CLINICIAN'S DESK REFERENCE

Diabetes

R David Leslie
MD, FRCP

Professor of Diabetes and Autoimmunity
and Consultant Physician,
St. Bartholomew's and Royal London Hospitals,
and the Blizard Institute, University of London

M Cecilia Lansang
MD, MPH

Co-chair, Diabetes Care Committee,
Cleveland Clinic,
Cleveland, Ohio

Simon Coppack
MD, FRCP

Consultant and Reader in Diabetes and Metabolism,
St. Bartholomew's and Royal London Hospitals,
and the Blizard Institute, University of London

Laurence Kennedy
MD, FRCP

Chairman, Department of Endocrinology, Diabetes,
and Metabolism,
Cleveland Clinic,
Cleveland, Ohio

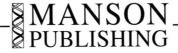

MANSON
PUBLISHING

Copyright © 2013 Manson Publishing Ltd

ISBN: 978-1-84076-158-0

A CIP catalogue record for this book is available from the British Library.

For full details of all Manson Publishing titles please write to:
Manson Publishing Ltd, 73 Corringham Road, London NW11 7DL, UK.
Tel: +44(0)20 8905 5150
Fax: +44(0)20 8201 9233
Website: www.mansonpublishing.com

Commissioning editor: Jill Northcott
Project manager: Ayala Kingsley
Copy editor: Joanna Brocklesby
Book and diagram design: Ayala Kingsley
Proof reader: John Forder
Indexer: Jill Dormon
Color reproduction: Tenon & Polert Colour Scanning Ltd, Hong Kong
Printed by: Butler Tanner & Dennis Ltd, Frome, Somerset, UK

Contents

Preface

THE AIM OF THIS BOOK is to provide clinicians and other health professionals with an easily readable and clinically applicable text on diabetes. The joint European and American authorship indicates the widespread international agreement on the best way to manage diabetes, both in terms of limiting the disease risk and of treating complications once they develop. The book integrates the physiology and anatomy of the disease with clinical and laboratory analysis. Summaries of key clinical trials emphasize the knowledge base underlying the practical recommendations. A range of treatment options is provided, reflecting the need for customized treatment strategies. The authors have sought to provide a clear and concise guide to the optimal treatment approach. The text is intended for clinicians with an interest in diabetes at all levels, including primary-care physicians, medical students, nurse specialists, physician assistants, diabetes educators, and those in postgraduate training.

R DAVID LESLIE
M CECILIA LANSANG
SIMON COPPACK
LAURENCE KENNEDY

Acknowledgments

Drs. Leslie, Coppack, and Kennedy would especially like to acknowledge the major role of their co-author, Dr. Lansang, in reviewing and updating the text during the gestation of this book.

We would all like to thank Professor David Hadden, Belfast, Northern Ireland, and Professor David Bell, Birmingham, Alabama, for providing constructive criticism and comments while we were preparing the text, and specifically acknowledge the valuable input of Professor Hadden concerning the most up-to-date views on diabetes and pregnancy.

We also thank Dr. Ernesto Lopez, Dr. Frida Djukiadmodjo, Dr. Lily Ho-Le, Dr. Serena Chiu, and Dr. Lina Paschou for their help in preparing and editing the text and figures.

In addition, the authors would like to thank Dr Michael Tolentino and Dr. Rishi Singh for supplying the retinal photos.

Abbreviations

AACE	American Association of Clinical Endocrinologists
ABX	abciximab
ACEI	angiotensin-converting enzyme inhibitor
acyl-CoA	acyl-coenzyme-A
ADA	American Diabetes Association
ADP	adenosine diphosphate
AGE	advanced glycation endproducts
AGI	a-glucosidase inhibitor
ALLHAT	Anti-Hypertensive and Lipid-Lowering Treatment to Prevent Heart Attacks Trials
AMPK	AMP-activated protein kinase
ARB	angiotensin-receptor blocker
ATP	adenosine triphosphate
AUC	area under the curve

BARI	Bypass Angioplasty Revascularization Investigation (trial)
BENEDICT	Bergamo Nephrologic Diabetes Complications Trial
BMI	body mass index
BP	blood pressure
BUN	blood urea nitrogen

C4	complement 4
CABG	coronary artery bypass grafting
CAD	coronary artery disease
cAMP	cyclic adenosine monophosphate
CAPD	continuous ambulatory peritoneal dialysis
CARDS	Collaborative Atorvastatin Diabetes Study
CARE	Cholesterol and Recurrent Events (trial)
CHF	congestive heart failure
CK-MB	creatine kinase, muscle–brain type
CNS	central nervous system
CRP	C-reactive protein
CSF	cerebrospinal fluid
CSII	continuous subcutaneous insulin infusion
CT	computed tomography
CVD	cardiovascular disease

DAN	diabetic autonomic neuropathy
DNA	deoxyribonucleic acid
DCCT	Diabetes Control and Complications Trial
DIGAMI	Diabetes Mellitus Insulin Glucose Infusion in Acute Myocardial Infarction (study)
DKA	diabetic ketoacidosis
DPP	Diabetes Prevention Program
DPP	dipeptidyl peptidase
DREAM	Diabetes REduction Assessment with ramipril and rosiglitazone Medication (trial)
DSME	diabetes self-management education
DVLA	Driver and Vehicle Licensing Agency

EASD	European Association for the Study of Diabetes
ECD	expanded criteria donor
ECG	electrocardiogram
ED50	effective dose of insulin that produces 50% of maximal effect
eGFR	estimated glomerular filtration rate
EGIR	European Group for the Study of Insulin Resistance
eNOS	endothelial nitric oxide synthase
EPIC	Evaluation of Platelet IIb/IIIa Inhibition for Prevention of Ischemic Complications (trial)
EPILOG	Evaluation of PTCA to Improve Long-term Outcome by c7E3 GP IIb/IIIa Receptor Blockade (trial)
EPISTENT	Evaluation of Platelet IIb/IIIa Inhibitor for Stenting (trial)
ESR	erythrocyte sedimentation rate
ESRD	end-stage renal disease
ETDRS	Early Treatment Diabetic Retinopathy Study

FDA	Food and Drug Administration
FEV1	forced expiratory volume in 1 second
FFA	free fatty acids
FIELD	Fenofibrate Intervention and Event Lowering in Diabetes (study)
FPG	fasting plasma glucose
FSH	follicle-stimulating hormone
FTO	fused-toe gene

GAD	glutamic acid decarboxylase
GADA	glutamic acid decarboxylase antibody
GBM	glomerular basement membrane
GDM	Gestational diabetes mellitus
GFAT	glutamine:fructose-6 phosphate amido-transferase
GFR	glomerular filtration rate
GIP	glucose-dependent insulinotrophic peptide
GIR	glucose infusion rate
GLP	glucagon-like peptide
GLUT	glucose transporter protein

HAPO	Hyperglycemia and Adverse Pregnancy Outcome (study)
HbA1c	glycated hemoglobin
HDL	high-density lipoprotein
HGO	hepatic glucose output
HLA	histocompatibility leukocyte antigen
H/Ma	hemorrhages or microaneurysms
HNF	hepatic nuclear factor
HONK	hyperosmolar nonketotic hyperglycemia
HOT	Hypertension Optimal Treatment (trial)
HHS	hyperosmolar hyperglycemic state

IAA	insulin autoantibody
IA-2	insulinoma-associated antigen-2
IADPSG	International Association of the Diabetes and Pregnancy Study Groups
IAPP	islet amyloid polypeptide
IDF	International Diabetes Federation
IDNT	Irbesartan Type 2 Diabetic Nephropathy Trial
IFCC	International Federation of Clinical Chemistry
IFG	impaired fasting glycemia
IGF	insulin-like growth factor
IgG	immunoglobulin G
IGT	impaired glucose tolerance
IPF-1	insulin promoter factor-1
IR	immunoreactive (insulin)
IRMA	intraretinal microvascular abnormalities
IRMA-2	Irbesartan in Patients with Type 2 Diabetes and Microalbuminuria (study)

KATP	ATP-sensitive potassium (channel)
K_m	Michaelis constant
KPD	ketosis-prone diabetes

LADA	latent autoimmune diabetes of adults
LDL	low-density lipoprotein
LDL-C	low-density lipoprotein cholesterol
LH	luteinizing hormone
LIFE	Losartan Intervention for Endpoint Reduction (study)
LIPID	Long-Term Intervention with Pravastatin in Ischemic Disease (trial)

MDI	multiple daily insulin injections
MDRD	Modification of Diet in Renal Disease (formula)
MHC	major histocompatibility complex
Micro-HOPE	Micro-Heart Outcomes Prevention Evaluation (study)
MODY	maturity onset diabetes of the young
MNT	medical nutrition therapy
MRFIT	Multiple Risk Factor Intervention Trial
MRI	magnetic resonance imaging

NAD	nicotinamide adenine dinucleotide
NADPH	nicotinamide adenine dinucleotide phosphate
NAVIGATOR	Nateglinide and Valsartan in Impaired Glucose Tolerance Outcomes Research (trial)
NCEP	National Cholesterol Education Program
NDDG	National Diabetes Data Group
NEFA	nonesterified fatty acids
NFκB	nuclear factor-kappa B
NICE	National Institute for Health and Clinical Excellence
NICE-SUGAR	Normoglycaemia in Intensive Care Evaluation and Survival Using Glucose Algorithm Regulation (study)
NIDDM	noninsulin-dependent diabetes mellitus
NIMGU	noninsulin-mediated glucose uptake
NPDR	nonproliferative diabetic retinopathy
NPH	neutral protamine Hagedorn
NVD	neovascularization near the optic disk
NVE	neovascularization elsewhere

OGTT	oral glucose tolerance test
OECD	Organisation for Economic Co-operation and Development
OHA	oral hypoglycemic agents

PARP	poly(ADP-ribose) polymerase		UDP	uridine diphosphate
PDE5	phosphodiesterase type-5		UGDP	University Group Diabetes Program
PDR	proliferative diabetic retinopathy		UKPDS	UK Prospective Diabetes Study
PKC	protein kinase C			
PKC-b	protein kinase C-beta		VA-HIT	Veterans Affairs HDL Intervention Trial
PPAR	peroxisome proliferator-activated receptor		VB	venous beading
			VCAM	vascular cell adhesion molecule
PTCA	percutaneous transluminal coronary angioplasty		VEGF	vascular endothelial growth factor
			VIP	vasoactive intestinal peptide
RAGE	advanced glycation endproduct receptor		VISEP	Efficacy of Volume Substitution and Insulin Therapy in Severe Sepsis (study)
RENAAL	Reduction of Endpoints in NIDDM with the Angiotensin II Antagonist Losartan (trial)		VLDL	very low-density lipoprotein
			VLDLR	very low density lipoprotein receptor
RIA	radio-immunoassay		VSMC	vascular smooth muscle cell
ROS	reactive oxygen species			
RNA	ribonucleic acid		WESDR	Wisconsin Epidemiologic Study of Diabetic Retinopathy
SGLT	sodium–glucose co-transporter		WHO	World Health Organization
SMBG	self-monitored blood glucose			
STOP-NIDDM	Study to Prevent NIDDM (trial)		XENDOS	XENical in the Prevention of Diabetes in Obese Subjects (study)
SU	sulfonylurea			
			ZnT8	zinc transporter 8
TRIPOD	Troglitazone in the Prevention of Diabetes (study)			
TZD	thiazolidinedione			

CHAPTER 1

The nature of diabetes

What is diabetes?

Overview

◆ Diabetes mellitus is a serious chronic hormonal condition in which the body is unable to properly use the energy from food.

◆ The name 'diabetes mellitus' differentiates the condition from the much rarer diabetes insipidus. Both of these conditions cause an increase in urine production; the urine in diabetes mellitus – but not diabetes insipidus – is sweet because of the glucose it contains. Diabetes mellitus will be referred to simply as diabetes in this book.

◆ Diabetes occurs when either the pancreas does not produce enough insulin (insulin deficiency) or the insulin is ineffective (insulin resistance). The function of insulin is to enable glucose to enter the body's cells in order to be used as energy. When glucose cannot enter the cells, its levels in the blood increase, resulting in hyperglycemia.

◆ The cause of diabetes is not known. Genetic and environmental factors both appear to be involved.

◆ There are two main types of diabetes:

◇ *Type 1* (insulin-dependent) diabetes, where the beta (β)-cells of the pancreas (**1**) are damaged so that little or no insulin is produced. This type is most often diagnosed in children or young adults. Patients with type 1 diabetes have to use injectable insulin to control blood glucose levels.

Diabetes occurs as a result of insulin deficiency and/or insulin resistance.

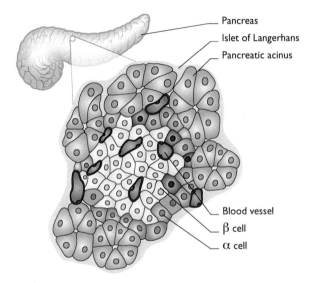

1 Beta cells. Beta cells contained within the islets of Langerhans produce the hormone insulin that controls glucose levels in the blood. Type 1 diabetes is caused by autoimmune destruction of these cells, while in type 2 diabetes their function deteriorates over time. Alpha cells produce glucagon – a counter-regulatory hormone.

◇ *Type 2* (noninsulin-dependent) diabetes, where some insulin is produced but is not fully taken up by the tissues. Type 2 diabetes is associated with obesity and is most commonly diagnosed in adults. This type of diabetes can be controlled with diet and exercise, and sometimes medication.

◇ These two types of diabetes differ in their pathogenesis and metabolic features.

◆ Long-term complications in blood vessels, kidneys, eyes, and nerves occur in both types of diabetes and are the major causes of morbidity and death.

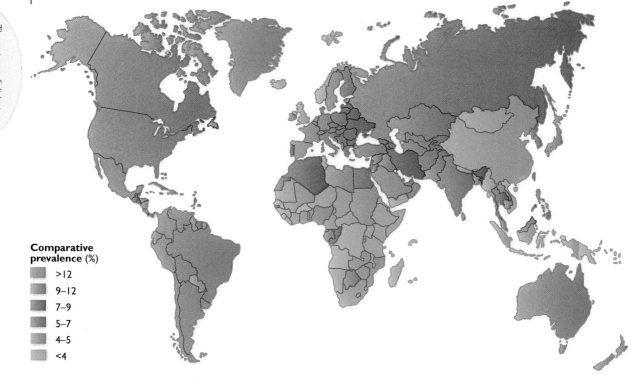

Comparative prevalence (%)

- >12
- 9–12
- 7–9
- 5–7
- 4–5
- <4

Epidemiology

◆ Diabetes is the most common metabolic disorder, with 5–10% of adult populations living affluent, westernized lifestyles developing the condition at some time in their life.

◆ According to the World Health Organization (WHO) estimate for 2000, there were 171 million adults with diabetes in the world (2.8%). In 2011 the International Diabetes Federation (IDF) set the figure at 366 million (8.3%); this is predicted to rise to 552 million (9.9%) by 2030.

◆ The rates of both type 1 and type 2 diabetes are increasing:

◇ With the epidemic of obesity in affluent societies, the burden of type 2 diabetes at all ages is increasing exponentially.

◇ The incidence of type 1 diabetes has also been increasing for many years for reasons that are much less apparent.

◆ There is a wide variation in the prevalence of diabetes worldwide, though people in developed countries, Europe and North America, have shown the highest prevalence. However, in the next 25 years, developing countries around these industrialized zones, such as Mexico, the Gulf States, India, and Russia, are likely to show a higher prevalence (**2**, **3**). The greatest increase is expected to be seen in India.

2 Comparative prevalence of diabetes in adults 20–79 years of age in 2010. The global prevalence of diabetes in 2010 was 6.6% of the adult population and, with the population set to rise, is projected to reach 9.9% by 2030. *Source: International Diabetes Federation.*

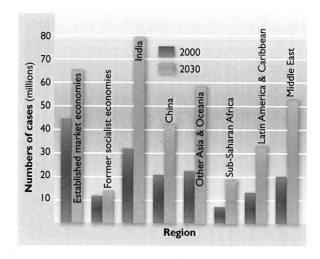

3 Regional changes. The greatest absolute increase in the number of people with diabetes by 2030 will likely be in India, with high relative increases also seen in the Middle East and sub-Saharan Africa.

It is estimated that the number of people with diabetes will more than triple between 2000 and 2030.

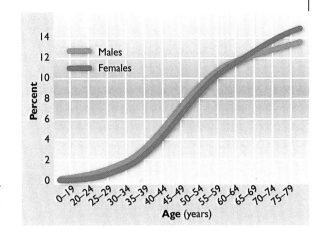

4 Diabetes prevalence by age and sex. Although diabetes prevalence is slightly higher in men than in women, the greater number of elderly women leads to a higher overall number of women with the disease.

- The predicted increase in incidence is, to a large extent, related to the increasing numbers of people living to more than 65 years of age. Diabetes is more prevalent in men, but there are more women than men with diabetes, as more women than men survive to old age in most societies (**4**).
- Figures for 2011 show the greatest number of people with diabetes to be in the 40–59 age group – 179 million; more than three-quarters of these people live in low- and middle-income countries.
  - ◇ By 2030, it is estimated that this number will increase to 250 million, with more than 86% living in low- and middle-income countries.
- Population screening programs typically reveal that up to half of the subjects found to have type 2 diabetes had previously been undiagnosed.
- It is currently estimated that 490,000 children under the age of 14 have type 1 diabetes.
- The incidence of type 2 diabetes in children is approaching that of type 1 diabetes, having been only around 2–4% prior to 1994, and is predicted to outstrip type 1 diabetes in about 2020 on current trends.
- A particularly high proportion of children with type 2 diabetes, typically presenting around the time of puberty, require insulin on presentation.
  - ◇ Whether this is due to the accelerator hypothesis ('double diabetes effect'), whereby an individual's risk (and age at onset) of contracting type 1 diabetes is increased by the prior existence of a predisposition to type 2 diabetes or insulin resistance, is not clear.

- It is difficult to obtain accurate figures for deaths related to diabetes, because people with diabetes most often die from cardiovascular and renal disease, and it is these that are recorded on death certificates. The excess adult mortality due to diabetes in 2011 was estimated by the IDF to be 4.6 million worldwide, 8.2% of global (all cause) mortality. This mortality rate ranged from 6% in Africa to 15.7% in North America.
  - ◇ It is considered that, worldwide, diabetes is the fifth most common cause of death.

Definitions and classification

- Diabetes mellitus is characterized by increased blood glucose concentrations.
  - ◇ Such glucose concentrations vary as a continuum in different people and so the definition of diabetes is somewhat arbitrary, but the cut-off points were chosen in relation to levels of glycemia associated with specific diabetic complications such as retinopathy.
- Historically we define diabetes by either a raised fasting glucose or a raised glucose following oral glucose challenge. Random glucose levels can also be used if the patient has symptoms typical of hyperglycemia, such as thirst and polyuria.
- The WHO defined diabetes mellitus in 1979 but the definition was updated in 2000 to reflect better understanding of 'milder' glucose intolerance and its impact on vascular disease.

Globally, diabetes is considered to be the fifth leading cause of death.

WHO diagnostic criteria

1 Symptoms of diabetes plus casual plasma glucose concentration of 11.1 mmol/l (200 mg/dl)
(*Casual is defined as any time of day without regard to time since last meal. Symptoms of diabetes include polyuria, polydipsia, and unexplained weight loss*)

OR

2 Fasting plasma glucose 7.0 mmol/l (126 mg/dl)
(*Fasting is defined as no caloric intake for at least 8 h*)

OR

3 2 h postload glucose 11.1 mmol/l (200 mg/dl) during an OGTT*
(*The test should be performed as described by WHO, using a glucose load containing the equivalent of 75 g anhydrous glucose dissolved in water. Not recommended for routine clinical use*)

6 **Diagnostic glucose values.** For epidemiological or population screening purposes, the fasting or 2 h value after 75 g oral glucose may be used alone. For clinical purposes, the diagnosis of diabetes should always be confirmed by repeating the test on another day, unless there is unequivocal hyperglycemia with acute metabolic decompensation or obvious symptoms. Glucose concentrations should not be determined on serum unless red cells are immediately removed, otherwise glycolysis will result in an unpredictable underestimation of the true concentrations. Note that glucose preservatives do not totally prevent glycolysis. If whole blood is used, the sample should be kept at 0–4°C or centrifuged/assayed immediately.

5 **Diagnostic criteria for diabetes.** In the absence of unequivocal hyperglycemia, these criteria should be confirmed by repeat testing on a different day. In 2011 the WHO accepted the use of the HbA1c test in diagnosing diabetes, with 48 mmol/mol (6.5%) recommended as the cut-off point.

◆ The WHO criteria for diagnosis are shown in **5** and **6**.
  ◇ WHO criteria only consider fasting and 120-min values in the oral glucose tolerance test (OGTT). Intermediate time points are used in the National Diabetes Data Group (NDDG) criteria.
  ◇ The reproducibility of the OGTT leaves much to be desired (the coefficient of variation of 120-min plasma glucose concentrations is reported to be up to 50%).
◆ Even if a subject fulfils the WHO criteria for diabetes, subsequent improvement in glucose tolerance can possibly occur (for example, as a result of weight loss or spontaneously), but such individuals are considered to have a lifelong tendency to diabetes.
◆ Impaired glucose tolerance (IGT) and impaired fasting glycemia (IFG) are metabolic states intermediate between normal glucose tolerance and diabetes mellitus (**6**). People with IFG or IGT are at high risk of progression to diabetes and/or cardiovascular disease.

Glucose concentration values (mmol/l [mg/dl])

		WHOLE BLOOD Venous	WHOLE BLOOD Capillary	PLASMA Venous
Diabetes mellitus	Fasting *or*	≥6.1 (≥110)	≥6.1 (≥110)	≥7.0 (≥126)
	2 h post-glucose load *or both*	≥10.0 (≥180)	≥11.1 (≥200)	≥11.1 (≥200)
Impaired glucose tolerance (IGT)	Fasting (if measured) *and*	<6.1 (<110)	<6.1 (<110)	<7.0 (<126)
	2 h post-glucose load	≥6.7 (≥120) *and* <10.0 (<180)	≥7.8 (≥140) *and* <11.1 (<200)	≥7.8 (≥140) *and* <11.1 (<200)
Impaired fasting glycemia (IFG)	Fasting	≥5.6 (≥100) *and* <6.1 (<110)	≥5.6 (≥100) *and* <6.1 (<110)	≥6.1 (≥110) *and* <7.0 (<126)
	and (if measured) 2 h post-glucose load	<6.7 (<120)	<7.8 (<140)	<7.8 (<140)

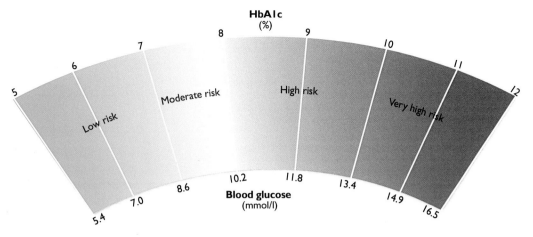

HbA1c
(%)

Blood glucose
(mmol/l)

Low risk

Moderate risk

High risk

Very high risk

Diabetes is characterized by hyperglycemia.

7 HbA1c and diabetes risk. The higher the HbA1c the higher the risk of diabetic complications.

- Diagnostic criteria based on glycated hemoglobin or hemoglobin A1c (HbA1c) have recently been proposed. Reflecting average glycemia over 2–3 months, this gives equal or almost equal sensitivity and specificity to glucose measurement.
  - ◇ HbA1c can be expressed as a percentage, as in the DCCT (Diabetes Control and Complications Trial). Alternatively it can be expressed as mmol/mol, which is recommended by the International Federation of Clinical Chemistry (IFCC) and is now the standard in the UK. A level of HbA1c of 6.0% (42 mmol/mol) or higher is considered abnormal by most laboratories and ≥6.5% (48 mmol/mol) broadly equates with the diagnosis of diabetes.
- Recent changes to the diagnostic criteria for diabetes reflect recognition of the increased cardiovascular risk evident at even modest levels of fasting hyperglycemia (~6.0 mmol/l or 100–110 mg/dl in some studies) (**7**).
  - ◇ However, the blood glucose threshold for cardiovascular effects is almost certainly lower than the threshold for the microvascular complications (nephropathy, retinopathy, neuropathy) unique to diabetes mellitus. Some people diagnosed as diabetic may not, therefore, suffer these microvascular complications, which have traditionally characterized the disease and determined its management.

- Diabetes represents a group of metabolic disorders, all of which are characterized by hyperglycemia. Type 1 diabetes is the most florid; type 2 diabetes is the most common.
  - ◇ The other forms, although less common, are important because they may need distinct therapy.
  - ◇ Some forms of diabetes are 'secondary' to another disease. Secondary diabetes accounts for barely 1–2% of all new cases.
- Type 1 diabetes (insulin-dependent diabetes mellitus) and type 2 diabetes (noninsulin-dependent diabetes mellitus) represent two distinct disease processes, but clinically this distinction can be unclear.
  - ◇ In normal physiology, increased insulin secretion usually compensates for reductions in insulin sensitivity. Decreased insulin sensitivity is a feature of both types of diabetes, but it is more severe in type 2 diabetes.
- Several classifications of diabetes have been proposed. The most widely used is that of the WHO/NDDG/ADA (**8**, next page). It should be recognized that unanimity in nomenclature has yet to be achieved, especially in the areas of gestational diabetes, diabetes related to pancreatitis, and tropical/malnutrition-related diabetes.

Etiological classification of diabetes

I TYPE 1 DIABETES
(β-cell destruction, usually leading to absolute insulin deficiency)

Immune-mediated
Idiopathic

II TYPE 2 DIABETES
(may range from predominantly insulin resistance with relative insulin deficiency
to a predominantly secretory defect with insulin resistance)

III OTHER SPECIFIC TYPES

Genetic defects of β-cell function	Chromosome 12, HNF-1α (MODY3) Chromosome 7, glucokinase (MODY2) Chromosome 20, HNF-4α (MODY1) Chromosome 13, insulin promoter factor-1 (IPF-1; MODY4) Chromosome 17, HNF-1α (MODY5) Chromosome 2, NeuroD1 (MODY6) Mitochondrial DNA Others	**Drug- or chemical-induced***	Vacor Pentamidine Nicotinic acid Glucocorticoids Thyroid hormone Diazoxide β-adrenergic agonists Thiazides Dilantin α-interferon Others
Genetic defects in insulin action	Type A insulin resistance Leprechaunism Rabson–Mendenhall syndrome Lipoatrophic diabetes Others	**Infections***	Congenital rubella Cytomegalovirus Others
Diseases of the exocrine pancreas*	Pancreatitis Trauma/pancreatectomy Neoplasia Cystic fibrosis Hemochromatosis Fibrocalculous pancreatopathy Others	**Uncommon forms of immune-mediated diabetes***	'Stiff-man' syndrome Anti-insulin receptor antibodies Others
Endocrinopathies*	Acromegaly Cushing's syndrome Glucagonoma Pheochromocytoma Hyperthyroidism Somatostatinoma Aldosteronoma Others	**Other genetic syndromes sometimes associated with diabetes**	Down's syndrome Klinefelter's syndrome Turner's syndrome Wolfram's syndrome Friedreich's ataxia Huntington's chorea Laurence–Moon–Biedl syndrome Myotonic dystrophy Porphyria Prader–Willi syndrome Others

IV GESTATIONAL DIABETES MELLITUS (GDM)
Statistical risk classes (subjects with normal glucose tolerance but substantially
increased risk of developing diabetes)

Previous abnormality of glucose tolerance
Potential abnormality of glucose tolerance

From WHO Study Group on Diabetes Mellitus
*Causes marked with an asterisk are termed 'secondary' diabetes.

8 Classification categories. There are four major categories of diabetes: type 1 diabetes and type 2 diabetes are the most common.

Forms of diabetes

Type 1 diabetes (see also chapter 3)

- Type 1 diabetes is the result of severe insulin deficiency leading to insulin-dependent diabetes. Though more commonly seen in those who develop diabetes during childhood or young adulthood, it can also occur at later ages.
  - ◇ In developed countries almost all patients have the immune-mediated form of the disease. This is an autoimmune disorder, where the body produces antibodies which destroy the insulin-producing cells of the pancreas. It is not clear what triggers this form of type 1 diabetes, but it is believed that both genetic and environmental factors (e.g. viruses) may be involved.
  - ◇ Idiopathic diabetes, where no cause can be found, is extremely rare.
- Type 1 diabetes is the second most common chronic disease of childhood after asthma.

9 Differential diagnosis. The distinction between the common types of diabetes and MODY is not always simple.

Type 2 diabetes (see also chapter 4)

- Type 2 diabetes occurs as a result of relative insulin deficiency, where the pancreas does not produce enough insulin, and insulin resistance, where the body's cells do not react normally to insulin. Type 2 diabetes is more prevalent than type 1 diabetes.
- The exact causes of type 2 diabetes are not understood, but risk factors include obesity, having a close relative with type 2 diabetes, being of south Asian, African–Caribbean or Middle Eastern descent, and being over 40 years of age. Though more common in adults, type 2 diabetes is increasing in incidence among children.

Maturity onset diabetes of the young (MODY)

- There have been several previous terms for this group of conditions. They are unified by being forms of diabetes mellitus with a strong family history and early onset, usually in children or adolescents. In the main, they do not present with ketosis and weight loss as in type 1 and there is no strong linkage with obesity as for type 2. MODY is a group of diabetic conditions distinct from type 1 and type 2 diabetes (**9**).

Differential diagnosis between diabetes types 1 and 2 and MODY

	TYPE 1 DIABETES	TYPE 2 DIABETES	MODY
Pathophysiology	β-cell failure	β-cell dysfunction and insulin resistance	β-cell dysfunction
Age of onset	Peak at 10–14 years old, but increasingly recognized in adults	Predominantly in middle to old age, but increasingly recognized in children	Typically childhood to young adulthood
Inheritance	Polygenic; heterogeneous	Polygenic; heterogeneous	Autosomal dominant
Role of environment	Considerable	Considerable	Minimal
Gender ratio	Males and females equally affected	Females affected more than males	Males and females equally affected
Association with obesity	<24% overweight	85% overweight	Uncommonly associated with obesity
Treatment required	Insulin required in >95%	Insulin required in 17–37% of children, but less frequent initially in adults	Insulin may be required but infrequently
Diabetes-specific autoantibodies status	Usually positive	Negative	Negative

- MODY is inherited in autosomal dominant fashion; there are several forms (**10**).
- MODY2 and MODY3 are due to defined insulin secretory defects.
- MODY should be considered in young people presenting with a typical family history (diabetes affecting a parent and 50% expression of the disease in the family).

I0 MODY subgroups. The clinical and genetic characteristics of the different subgroups are outlined. Frequency and penetrance are most pronounced with MODY3.

Gestational diabetes mellitus (GDM)
(see also chapter 15)

- GDM occurs when abnormal glucose tolerance develops during pregnancy in a woman not known to have diabetes before pregnancy, unless she has had GDM in a previous pregnancy.
- The abnormal glucose tolerance usually resolves after delivery, but women with GDM are quite likely to develop it again in a subsequent pregnancy, and are at considerably increased risk of developing type 2 diabetes some time in the future.

Characteristics of MODY subgroups

	MODY1	MODY2	MODY3	MODY4	MODY5	MODY-X
Frequency (%)	2	30	64	<1	2	12
Genetics	HNF-4α (20q13)	Glucokinase (7p15)	HNF-1α (12q24)	IPF-1 (13q12)	HNF-1β, (17cen-q21)	NeuroD1 (β2)
Penetrance of mutations at 40 years of age (%)	>80	45 (>90% with FPG>6 mmol/l)	>95	>80	>95	Not known
Pathophysiology	β-cell dysfunction (glucose sensing)	β-cell dysfunction	β-cell dysfunction (sulfonylurea sensitive)	β-cell dysfunction	β-cell dysfunction	β–cell dysfunction
Onset of hyperglycemia	Adolescence, early adulthood (12–35 years)	Early childhood (from birth)	Adolescence, early adulthood (12–28 years)	Adolescence, early adulthood (14–40 years)	Adolescence, early adulthood (12–28 years)	> 40years of age
Severity of hyperglycemia	Progressive IGT (may become severe)	Mild, stable hyperglycemia; little deterioration with age	Progressive IGT (may be severe)	Progressive IGT (may become severe)	Progressive IGT (may be severe)	Variable
Microvascular complications	Can occur	Rare	Can occur	Can occur	Especially renal	Variable
Treatment	Usually sulfonylureas; occasionally insulin	Diet and exercise	Usually diet alone or sulfonylureas	Usually sulfonylureas; occasionally insulin	Usually insulin	Usually insulin
Other features		Reduced birth weight	Low renal threshold	Pancreatic agenesis in homozygotes	Renal cysts, proteinuria, renal failure	

FPG, fasting plasma glucose; HNF, hepatic nuclear factor; IGT, impaired glucose tolerance; IPF, insulin promoter factor; NeuroD1, neurogenic differentiation 1.

- Risk factors for GDM include obesity, older age, first-degree relatives with diabetes, a history of poor pregnancy outcome, a history of large for gestational age babies, and belonging to an ethnic/racial group with a known high prevalence of type 2 diabetes.

Neonatal diabetes

- Neonatal diabetes develops in neonates shortly after birth and within the first 2 years of life. It can be transient or permanent. It is due to a defect in the potassium channel of insulin-secreting cells, as a result of gene mutations which limit potassium channel closure and thus insulin secretion.
- The gene mutations can be rectified by sulfonylureas which enable activation of the potassium channel, so that children treated with insulin can switch to sulfonylurea treatment with an improvement in glucose control.

Secondary diabetes

- This book is not intended to be an authoritative account of the diagnosis and management of the multiple conditions that may cause secondary diabetes or glucose intolerance. Such conditions are listed in **8**.

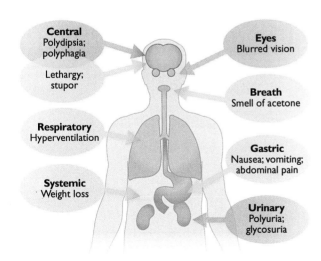

- Patients with diabetes present either with symptoms due to the high glucose level or with the complications of diabetes (**11**).
- The classic triad of symptoms directly due to high blood glucose is:
  - ◇ Polyuria – due to the osmotic diuresis that results when blood glucose levels exceed the renal threshold.
  - ◇ Thirst – due to the resulting loss of fluid and electrolytes.
  - ◇ Weight loss – due to fluid depletion and the accelerated breakdown of fat and muscle secondary to insulin deficiency; this is less prevalent in those with type 2 diabetes.
- Florid symptoms are most often seen in children with type 1 diabetes. Ketoacidosis may be a presenting feature.
- Patients with type 1 diabetes often, but not always, present with severe symptoms of hyperglycemia.
  - ◇ The severity of the condition may be reflected in raised blood ketone levels and weight loss.
- Other, nonosmotic symptoms are the consequences of high blood glucose:
  - ◇ Lack of energy.
  - ◇ Visual blurring (due to glucose-induced changes in refraction).
  - ◇ Fungal infections causing pruritus vulvae and balanitis.
  - ◇ Bacterial infections causing staphylococcal skin infections.
  - ◇ Retinopathy.
  - ◇ Polyneuropathy causing tingling and numbness in the feet or erectile dysfunction.

11 Symptoms of diabetes. Those symptoms in orange are typically confined to patients with type 1 diabetes.

The classic symptoms directly due to hyperglycemia are polyuria, thirst, and weight loss.

◆ Subjects with IGT are at risk of macrovascular disease and some already have arterial disease on presentation, including myocardial infarction and gangrene.

◆ A fraction of cases present without symptoms, either on routine blood screening or with glycosuria.

  ◇ Glycosuria is not diagnostic of diabetes but indicates the need for further investigation.

  ◇ About 1% of the population have renal glycosuria, inherited as an autosomal dominant or recessive trait associated with a low renal threshold for glucose.

◆ As a common disease that can have multiple consequences, diabetes may be discovered 'fortuitously' in patients being investigated for a wide range of symptoms.

Complications of diabetes

◆ If diabetes is not well managed or controlled, the high blood glucose levels can lead to damage to blood vessels, nerves, and organs. Even non-symptomatic, mild hyperglycemia can have damaging effects in the long term. High blood sugar levels can also reduce the efficiency of white blood cells in fighting infections.

Macrovascular complications
(see also Chapter 6)

◆ Macrovascular problems associated with diabetes mellitus include heart disease, stroke, and peripheral vascular disease (which can lead to ulcers, gangrene, and amputation). Prolonged, poorly controlled hyperglycemia increases the likelihood of atherosclerosis. An individual with diabetes is approximately five times more likely to suffer heart disease and stroke than someone without diabetes.

Diabetes dramatically increases an individual's risk of heart disease and stroke.

Microvascular complications

◆ These include retinopathy, neuropathy, and nephropathy (see also Chapters 6, 7, 8, 9, 10).

◆ Very small blood vessels can become blocked or leaky as a result of hyperglycemia. The blood vessels most frequently affected are in the eye, the kidney, and nerve sheaths. This microvascular disease is specific to diabetes, and may occur in any type of diabetes.

  ◇ Damage to the blood vessels of the retina can result in loss of vision.

  ◇ Damage to blood vessels in the kidneys can result in kidney failure.

  ◇ Damage to blood vessels in nerve sheaths can result in numbness or tingling. If nerves to the digestive system are affected, the individual may suffer associated symptoms, e.g. nausea or constipation. Loss of sensation in the feet can lead to the development of ulcers.

Acute metabolic complications

◆ These include hypoglycemia, ketoacidosis, hyperosmolar nonketotic hyperglycemia (see also Chapter 11).

◆ Hypoglycemia most commonly results from treating diabetes with exogenous insulin or insulin secretagogues.

  ◇ In a person without diabetes, endogenous production of insulin decreases and counter-regulatory hormones (mostly epinephrine and glucagon) increase, in response to hypoglycemia. This fine-tuned system is dysregulated in patients with diabetes, and patients have to resort to intake of carbohydrates to raise the blood glucose back up to normal.

  ◇ Symptoms range from mild to moderate (palpitations, diaphoresis) to severe (convulsions, coma).

◆ Diabetic ketoacidosis and hyperosmolar hyperglycemic nonketotic state occur as a result of insulin deficiency during episodes of stress, when counter-regulatory hormones are in excess.

  ◇ Patients are dehydrated, and frequently present with altered sensorium. Treatment includes hydration to correct the fluid deficit, insulin administration, and correction of the underlying disease.

Common infections

Staphylococcal infections (boils, abscesses, carbuncles)
Fungal infections (mouth, nails, skin folds)
Mucocutaneous candidiasis
Chronic peridontitis
Urinary tract infections
Pyelonephritis
Staphylococcal and pneumococcal pneumonia
Tuberculosis

12 Common infections. Damage to nerves and blood vessels, as well as high blood-sugar levels, increases the diabetic patient's vulnerability to infection.

Infections

◆ Diabetic patients are prone to a range of different infections including bacterial, tuberculosis, and fungal (**12**). Several factors lead to this predisposition:

◇ The integrity of the skin barrier is often disrupted in diabetic patients as a result of neuropathy, with dry cracking skin or otherwise loss of protective sensation. Cellulitis often results from this.

◇ The impaired vascularity, thus reduced oxygen and nutrient delivery to the periphery, predisposes to infections and also results in poor antibiotic delivery.

◇ Hyperglycemia can affect the immune response, resulting in impaired phagocytosis and chemotaxis as well as decreased antibody function. Allied to problems with blood supply and maintaining the skin surface structure, this probably explains the excess risk of this broad range of infections.

◆ Conversely, infections may lead to loss of glycemic control, and are a common cause of ketoacidosis and hyperosmolar nonketotic hyperglycemia.

◇ Insulin-treated patients need to increase their dose in the face of infection, and noninsulin-treated patients may need insulin therapy when they have an infection.

◆ Diabetes is associated with a number of life-threatening infections (**13**).

◇ Malignant otitis externa, when untreated, is associated with > 50% mortality, especially in patients who sustain facial nerve palsy.

◇ Rhinocerebral mucormycosis is particularly seen in those with diabetic ketoacidosis. The infection starts in the nose and paranasal sinuses, then spreads to the orbits, the cribriform plate, meninges, and brain.

◇ Emphysematous cholecystitis has a mortality rate at least triple that of acute cholecystitis, with perforation and gangrene being frequent.

13 Life-threatening infections. Several head, neck, pulmonary, and soft-tissue infections present a particular threat to diabetic patients.

Life-threatening infections in diabetic patients

TYPE	CAUSATIVE FACTORS	TREATMENT	MORTALITY (%)
Malignant otitis externa	*Pseudomonas aeruginosa*	Carbenicillin	10–20
Rhinocerebral mucormycosis	Fungi of the order Mucorales including *Rhizopus* and *Mucor* spp.	Amphotericin B	34
Emphysematous cholecystitis	*Clostridia* spp. or *Escherichia coli*	Ampicillin/clindamycin	15
Emphysematous pyelonephritis	*Escherichia coli* and other	Cephalosporin	10–37
Necrotizing fasciitis/cellulitis	Mixed aerobic	Imipenem	20
Nonclostridial gas gangrene	Mixed aerobic	Imipenem, debridement, hyperbaric oxygen	25–50

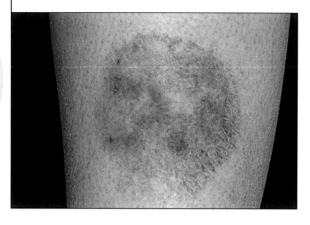

14 Necrobiosis lipoidica. Erythematous, atrophic plaque.

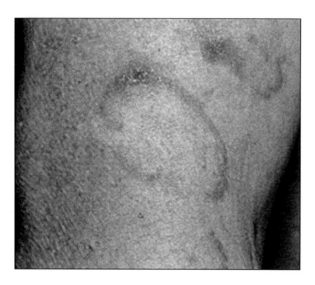

15 Granuloma annulare. Annular lesions of localized granuloma annulare.

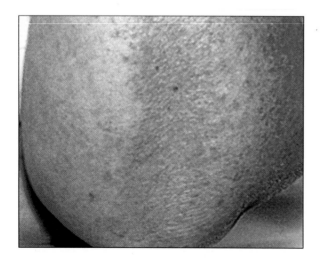

16 Granuloma annulare. Confluent plaque extensor surface of elbow in generalized granuloma annulare.

Several dermatopathies are directly related to diabetes.

Disorders of the joints, ligaments, and skin

◆ Glycation of ligaments is increased in diabetes. As a result, the ligaments of the hands and elsewhere are thickened and stiffened, limiting joint flexibility and promoting joint contractures.

  ◇ Stiffness of the hands with thick waxy skin, the diabetic hand or diabetic cheiroarthropathy, is especially common in childhood-onset diabetes. Cheiroarthropathy can be illustrated by the 'prayer sign', in which the patient opposes the hands as if in prayer; but the metacarpophalangeal and interphalangeal joints cannot be opposed.

◆ Rotator cuff syndrome of the shoulders is also more prevalent in diabetes.

◆ Osteopenia in the extremities has been described and may be a result of peripheral neuropathy.

◆ Acanthosis nigricans is a feature of insulin resistance, and is commonly seen in obese individuals.

  ◇ It appears as a velvety blackish or dark brown hyperkeratosis, most commonly on the nape, sides of the neck, axillae, and groin.

  ◇ It is a marker of hyperinsulinemia.

  ◇ There is no definitive treatment, but improvement has been seen in obese individuals who have lost weight.

◆ Necrobiosis lipoidica diabeticorum is commonly seen on the shins of diabetic patients, and occurs in the 3rd to 4th decades of life. However, it can also manifest in nondiabetic patients, and the shortened term necrobiosis lipoidica is sometimes preferred.

  ◇ It is usually seen as reddish-brown or brownish-purple plaques that slowly enlarge, later becoming yellowish in the center. The overlying epidermis becomes atrophic, leading to a shiny appearance and prominence of underlying blood vessels (**14**).

  ◇ Topical applications, intralesional injections of corticosteroids as well as various drugs (e.g. aspirin and nicotinamide) have been tried without clear evidence of benefit.

- Granuloma annulare is a benign asymptomatic dermatosis consisting of one or more localized annular lesions composed of a peripheral ring of papules with a flat central portion (**15**, **16**).
  - ◇ Granuloma annulare is usually found on the extremities, arms more than legs, in the young more than the old, and they rarely ulcerate. In contrast to necrobiosis it can presage diabetes, but as with necrobiosis there is no treatment.
- Lipoatrophy was more commonly seen with the use of the earlier insulin preparations, however it can still be seen in patients using human insulin or even insulin analogs. Local immune complex formation and complement fixation with lysosomal enzyme release have been implicated as the mechanisms for its development.
- Lipohypertrophy continues to be a complication, and is thought to be due to a local anabolic effect of insulin. The hypertrophic areas usually subside when insulin injections are rotated and these problematic sites are avoided. Patients are also advised not to use these areas for insulin injection because of the unpredictable absorption of insulin.
- Diabetic dermopathy is represented by mutiple, bilateral, pretibial, circumscribed, shallow scars and is the most common diabetic cutaneous condition especially associated with poor diabetes control. There is no treatment.
- Diabetic bullae are rare distinct features presenting with acute blistering of the extremeties which heal spontaneously.
- Diabetic nodular prurigo is characterized by inflamed, severely pruritic, nodular lesions predominantly on the extremeties, which form brown discolored plaques as they resolve.
  - ◇ Treatment is with steroid creams and antipruritic agents, as well as drugs used in diabetic neuritis such as tricyclic antidepressants. Nodular prurigo is usually associated with poor diabetes control which should be managed appropriately.

Type 2 diabetes accounts for 5% of the total healthcare costs in Europe.

The cost of diabetes

- The cost of diabetes is substantial and increasing as the cost of therapies rises and the disease frequency increases.
- There is a strong commercial argument, quite apart from a humanitarian one, for primary prevention of diabetes complications.
  - ◇ The cost of effectively treating the complications of diabetes is high, and preventive care in limiting progression to diabetic complications has a definite impact.
- There are striking differences in cost estimates between different countries. Most studies have shown that indirect costs (loss of financial output through illness or death, etc.) approximately equal direct costs (treatment, diagnosis, medical care, etc.). Management of diabetes only accounts for about 25% of the direct costs, the remainder being accounted for by long-term diabetic complications.
- Direct costs in the US alone for diabetes care rose from $1 billion in 1969 to $44.1 billion by 1992. The total estimated cost of diabetes in the US in 2007 is $174 billion, with direct medical costs amounting to $116 billion (**17**).
- Type 2 diabetes is not only the most prevalent form of diabetes, it also accounts for about 90% of the resources of diabetes care and about 5% of the total healthcare costs in Europe.

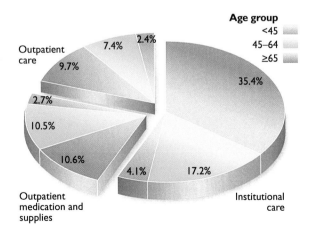

17 The cost of diabetes. Healthcare expenditures attributed to diabetes in the USA, by age group and type of service, 2007. Direct medical costs were $116 billion.

CHAPTER 2

Glucose, insulin, and diabetes

The role of glucose

◆ Glucose is a vital metabolic fuel, being the main source of energy in many tissues. It is metabolized during the process of cellular respiration, which breaks it down to release adenosine triphosphate (ATP).

◇ It is a monosaccharide, or simple sugar, with the formula $C_6H_{12}O_6$. Its six carbon atoms can be arranged in open-chain or ring forms.

◇ Red blood cells and brain cells use glucose almost exclusively for energy production, whereas other cells in the body can metabolize fats for energy if necessary.

◇ Most glucose in the body comes from digested carbohydrates, but it can also be synthesized in the liver.

◆ The importance of glucose is reflected in the strict control of blood glucose levels (homeostasis [**18**]). This contrasts with the relative laxity of regulation of other circulating metabolic fuels such as ketone bodies and nonesterified fatty acids (NEFA) (also known as free fatty acids [FFA]) – the form in which stored body fat is transported from adipose tissue to its sites of utilization.

◆ Of all the hormones known to influence blood glucose concentration, insulin is the only one able to lower it, implying the potential danger of lack of this fuel when the blood glucose is low (hypoglycemia).

◆ Glucose is also important in the formation of glycoproteins, making up the carbohydrate groups on proteins which play key roles in the normal functioning of enzymes and in protein binding.

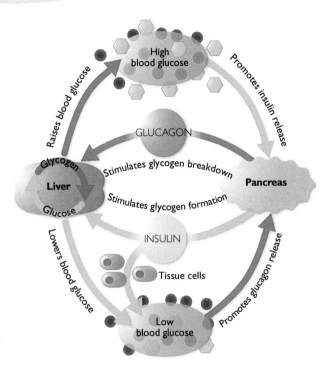

18 Glucose homeostasis. The concentration of glucose in the blood is controlled by the antagonistic actions of two hormones: insulin and glucagon, produced in the β cells and α cells of the pancreatic islets, respectively. High blood glucose causes the pancreas to release more insulin and less glucagon; the excess glucose is converted to glycogen and stored in the liver. If glucose levels are low, then the pancreas releases more glucagon and less insulin, stimulating the breakdown of glycogen back to glucose, which re-enters the bloodstream.

Glucose is the main source of energy for human body cells.

Insulin is the only hormone able to lower blood glucose concentration.

---

19 Postprandial metabolic responses. Insulin, glucose and NEFA concentrations in normal and obese subjects eating three meals a day (arrows). Normal insulin response to meals is rapid and relatively short-lasting. As the the insulin concentration rises in response to a meal, NEFA response is suppressed. Insulin resistance in obese individuals means that higher insulin levels are required to maintain normoglycemia. *Adapted from Reaven 1985.*

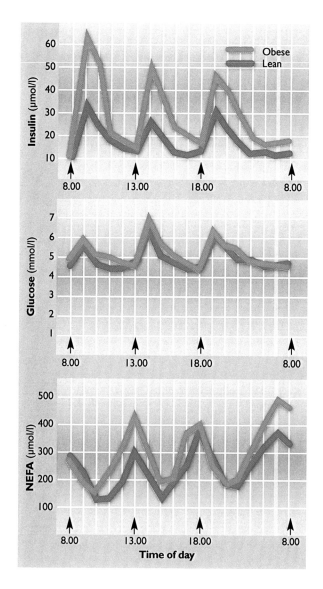

Glucose levels and diabetes

◆ Diabetes is defined by an increase in blood glucose levels above normal values. To understand how hyperglycemia may occur, we should consider factors that maintain blood glucose within a strict range.

◆ In healthy people, blood glucose concentrations are maintained within very close limits (**19**), with a strictly maintained postabsorptive (e.g. fasted overnight) blood glucose concentration of 4.5–5.2 mmol/l (81–94 mg/dl).

  ◇ Inter-individual coefficients of variation (assuming similar times since previous meal, meal composition, levels of activity, etc.) are <5%, so a fasting glucose of 6.0 mmol/l (108 mg/dl) is 4–5 standard deviations above the mean in most healthy populations.

  ◇ Glucose concentrations increase after meals, but typical meals will not raise blood glucose above ~8 mmol/l (144 mg/dl), and normoglycemia is usually restored within 2–4 hours in healthy people.

  ◇ Reductions in glycemia can be produced by severe, sudden, unaccustomed exercise or prolonged fasting (or both), by various pathological conditions (usually hepatic or gastroenterological) and by pharmacological means, but are not commonly encountered in healthy adults in developed countries.

◆ Strict avoidance of low blood sugars is necessary to avoid the neurological and other consequences of hypoglycemia (see also p. 168).

  ◇ Neuroglycopenia (glucose depletion in neural tissue) starts at concentrations around 3.0–3.5 mmol/l (54–63 mg/dl) and counter-regulatory mechanisms are set to respond to maintain glycemia comfortably above this level.

◆ The reason for the strict avoidance of hyperglycemia is less immediately apparent.

  ◇ Symptoms of hyperglycemia are florid (in subjects used to relative normoglycemia) at blood glucose concentrations of 12–13 mmol/l (216–234 mg/dl) and may commence at concentrations below 10 mmol/l (180 mg/dl). The metabolic consequences of severe hyperglycemia, at levels usually above 20 mmol/l (360 mg/dl), are discussed in the section on diabetic emergencies (p. 121).

◇ In contrast, mild hyperglycemia (glucose 6–9 mmol/l [108–162 mg/dl]) is usually asymptomatic. The value of the strict avoidance of mild hyperglycemia is thus not so apparent, except in terms of avoiding the consequences of prolonged hyperglycemia: long-term diabetic complications or tissue damage.

◇ Increased susceptibility to infection may be seen acutely with moderate hyperglycemia.

Normal glucose metabolism

◆ Glucose enters the circulation from three main sources:

◇ The gut, as the result of hydrolysis, or hepatic conversion of a variety of ingested carbohydrates.

◇ Hepatic and other glycogen stores (glycogenolysis).

◇ New synthesis from precursors (gluconeogenesis) (**20**).

20 Gluconeogenesis and glycogenolysis. Gluconeogenesis is the synthesis of glucose in the liver from noncarbohydrate sources, including lactic acid from the muscles. In glycogenolysis, glycogen reserves in the liver and muscles are converted back into glucose-6-phosphate to begin the glycolytic process, the end results of which are pyruvic acid and, via the citric acid cycle, ATP.

◆ *Gluconeogenesis* takes place in the liver (~75–90%) and kidneys (~10–25%).

◇ The breakdown of fat (from glycerol), muscle glycogen (from lactate), and amino acids (such as alanine), creates two 3-carbon molecules which combine to form the 6-carbon glucose molecule.

◇ In the resting postabsorptive state, hepatic glucose output is ~2.0 mg/kg bodyweight/min or 200–300 g during the average day (depending on the availability of glucose from food and the body's requirements).

◇ Glycemia is determined by the balance of glucose influx into the circulation (principally from hepatic glucose production) and peripheral clearance.

◆ *Glycogenesis* converts excess glucose into glycogen, via glucose-6-phosphate, for storage in the liver and muscles, while *glycogenolysis* is the process by which it is converted back again.

◇ Glycogen is synthesized from both glucose and the gluconeogenic precursors.

◇ A 70 kg man typically has a total of 700–1000 g of (hydrated) glycogen, mostly stored in the liver (60–125 g) and skeletal muscle (400–600 g).

◇ Glycogen in skeletal muscle can provide local fuel but does not provide a source of glucose for release into the circulation.

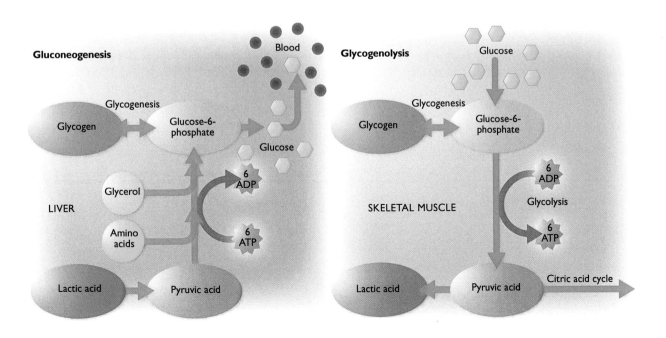

◆ *Glucose homeostasis* is accomplished predominantly by the liver, which absorbs and stores glucose (as glycogen) in the postabsorptive state and releases it into the circulation between meals.
  ◇ To maintain homeostasis, the rate of glucose utilization by peripheral tissues must match the rate of glucose production.
  ◇ The balancing of glucose production and utilization depends partly upon mass action, but also crucially upon endocrine regulation by insulin and its counter-regulatory hormones (see **18**).

◆ Glucose provides approximately 40–60% (on a typical western diet) of the total fuel expenditure of the body during a 24-hour period.
  ◇ It provides almost all the energy of the central nervous system.
  ◇ During high-intensity exercise and during the 4–6 hours postprandially, glucose is the predominant fuel of the whole body.
  ◇ Glucose is the most efficient fuel for oxidation in terms of the liberation of energy (112.2 kcal or 6 mole ATP per mole of oxygen consumed).
  ◇ Many tissues can use ketone bodies, fatty acids, or glucose for their energy supply, depending upon their relative availability in the circulation.

◆ Glucose is fully oxidized to carbon dioxide and water in the brain, liver, skeletal muscle, and some other tissues.
  ◇ The brain accounts for most of the glucose oxidized in the fasting state (100–125 g/24 h).
  ◇ In the fasted state, resting skeletal muscle takes up 10–20% of hepatic glucose output: this is not all oxidized but can be converted to lactate, pyruvate, glycerol, or amino acids, some of which subsequently returns to the liver as gluconeogenic precursors.
  ◇ Fatty acids (or their partial oxidation products, ketone bodies) are the major fuel of resting muscle, heart, and liver.
  ◇ Other tissues such as red blood cells, skin, adipose tissue, and the renal medulla derive most energy from glycolysis to lactate and pyruvate. Glycolysis to lactate is an anaerobic process to which many cells may resort when faced with hypoxia: for example, skeletal muscle during high-intensity exercise.

◇ Glucose taken up by fat tissue is used as a source of energy and to form the glycerol component of triglyceride stores.

◆ In resting, postabsorptive subjects, approximately 70% of the body's glucose metabolism occurs independently of the action of insulin. However, these insulin-independent mechanisms cannot maintain normoglycemia for very long.

◆ Insulin-independent (as well as insulin-dependent) glucose clearance is impaired in subjects with type 2 diabetes and also in normoglycemic subjects with a family history of diabetes. This suggests that abnormalities in insulin-independent glucose disposal manifest at a very early stage of disease evolution.
  ◇ This phenomenon of 'glucose resistance' appears to be quantitatively important: as much as half an intravenous glucose load is cleared by virtue of the effect of hyperglycemia on insulin-independent glucose disposal in normal subjects.

Glucose transporters

◆ Glucose is a hydrophilic molecule unable to penetrate the lipid bilayer of cell membranes.
  ◇ Its uptake into cells is achieved by an energy-independent process of facilitated diffusion mediated by a family of glucose transporter proteins (GLUTs).
  ◇ GLUT transporters allow the uptake of glucose into cells from the interstitial fluid into which glucose diffuses from the bloodstream. Differences in kinetics, tissue and subcellular expression profiles, and substrate specificities enable specific functions such as glucose sensing (GLUT2) and insulin-dependent glucose uptake (GLUT4) (**21**).

◆ The various sugar transporters recognized to date are classified into those having high glucose affinity (class I, comprising GLUT1–4), high fructose affinity (class II, e.g. GLUT5), and novel transporters whose physiology is not yet fully understood (GLUT6–14).

The entry of glucose into cells is mediated by a group of transporter proteins known as GLUTs.

Characteristics of the main glucose transporters

TRANSPORTER	TISSUES	KINETICS	TRANSPORT TYPE
GLUT1	Ubiquitous, erythrocyte, placenta, colon, kidney	Low K_m (~2 mmol/l, 18–36 mg/dl)	Facilitated diffusion
GLUT2	Liver, small intestine, kidney, β cells	High K_m (~20 mmol/l, 450 mg/dl), high V_{max}	Facilitated diffusion, bidirectional
GLUT3	Ubiquitous, brain, placenta, kidney	Low K_m (~1 mmol/l, 18–36 mg/dl), low V_{max} (6–7 mmol/l, 108–126 mg/dl)	Facilitated diffusion
GLUT4	Skeletal muscle, adipocyte, heart	K_m ~5 mmol/l (36–180 mg/dl)	Facilitated diffusion, insulin responsive
GLUT5	Jejunum		Facilitated diffusion of fructose
Na^+-glucose co-transporter(s)	Intestine, kidney tubules	Moves glucose against concentration gradient	Active transport, symport using Na^+ gradient

Glucose, insulin, and diabetes

21 Glucose transporter proteins. GLUT family members are tissue-specific. In addition, their differing kinetic properties allow a range of functions.

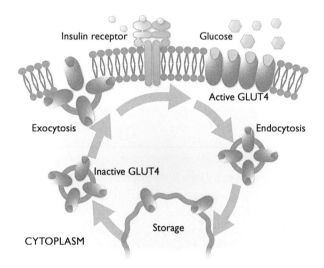

- The different functions of the class I GLUTs are related to their differing K_m values (K_m, the Michaelis constant, is the substrate concentration that produces half the maximum enzyme/transporter activity).
  - GLUT1, GLUT3, and GLUT4 have K_m values of approximately 1–5 mmol/l (36–90 mg/dl) but GLUT2 has a K_m value of approximately 20 mmol/l (450 mg/dl). This variation in K_m permits high rates of glucose entry into essential cells (e.g. central nervous system) even during relative hypoglycemia, via the low-K_m GLUT3, but at the same time permits the pancreatic β cells to sense increments in blood glucose over a range well exceeding normality via the high-K_m GLUT2.
  - The central nervous system is relatively protected from neuroglycopenia by the low K_m of its GLUT3 transporters.
- GLUT1 and GLUT3 transporters are present in the cell membrane at all times and allow cells to take up glucose independently of insulin action (a process sometimes termed noninsulin-mediated glucose uptake, NIMGU).

22 Insulin-dependent glucose uptake. When insulin is present, or there is muscle activity, GLUT4 molecules move from storage within the cell to the plasma membrane, where they contribute to glucose transport.

- In contrast, GLUT4 transporters are stored in the cell cytoplasm. In the presence of insulin, GLUT4 moves from these storage compartments to the cell membrane, increasing transporter numbers 6–10-fold. When insulin concentrations decline, GLUT4 is removed from the cell membrane by endocytosis and rapidly recycled back into storage (**22**).

- Dysfunction of the insulin-regulated GLUT4 translocation process appears to play a part in insulin resistance, and mutations of several transporters (e.g. GLUT1, GLUT2) have been associated with inborn errors of carbohydrate metabolism.
  - ◇ The insulin-sensitizing agents metformin and the thiazolidinediones appear to increase cell surface expression of GLUT4, as does physical exercise.
- Glucose can be moved against a concentration gradient – necessary in the special circumstances of the renal tubule and intestinal epithelium – by using a family of at least three known sodium–glucose co-transporters (SGLTs).
  - ◇ At least one of these co-transporters (SGLT3) appears to have some glucose concentration-sensing function.
  - ◇ Mutations of SGLT1 are associated with the glucose–galactose malabsorption syndrome, which can cause fatal infantile diarrhea unless these sugars are removed from the diet.
  - ◇ A reduced function mutation of SGLT2 has been associated with renal tubular glucose spillage.
- To trap glucose within the cell (since GLUTs are potentially bidirectional), glucose is phosphorylated on entry by a family of hexokinases.
  - ◇ Hexokinase types I–III are expressed widely and have low K_m.
  - ◇ Hexokinase type IV (also called glucokinase and predominantly expressed in liver and β cells) has a much higher K_m of up to 15 mmol/l (270 mg/dl), permitting it to function as a glucose sensor beyond the physiological range of blood glucose.
  - ◇ Since glucokinase action is also a rate-limiting step in glucose metabolism, it thus becomes a crucial determinant of the rate of insulin secretion from β cells.
- Loss-of-function mutations of glucokinase are responsible for one form of maturity onset diabetes of the young (MODY 2) (see p.18).

- Dephosphorylation of glucose (the reverse reaction) is catalyzed by glucose-6-phosphatase. This process is required for the export of glucose (from gluconeogenesis) by hepatic and renal cells in hypoinsulinemic situations.
  - ◇ Overactivity of glucose-6-phosphatase contributes to the increased and relatively insulin-insensitive hepatic glucose production in type 2 diabetes.
  - ◇ Metformin and the thiazolidinediones (see Chapter 13) appear to reduce the activity of this enzyme, although it is not clear whether their effects are direct or mediated through some other upstream action.

The role of insulin

- Insulin is the predominant hormone regulating blood glucose concentration. It is the key hormone involved in both the storage and the controlled release of energy.
- Diabetes occurs as a result of a failure of insulin production and secretion (insulin deficiency) and/or the loss of response to insulin (insulin resistance).
- Insulin is coded for by genes on chromosome 11 and is synthesized and secreted by the β cells of the islets of Langerhans in the pancreas. Complex cellular events trigger the release of insulin from the secretory granules of these cells.
- After secretion, insulin enters the portal circulation, which takes it to the liver, a prime target organ of insulin action.
- Although insulin is the major regulator of intermediary metabolism, its actions are modified by other hormones, e.g. glucagon, epinephrine (adrenalin), cortisol, and growth hormone. Such counter-regulatory hormones increase glucose production from the liver and, for a given level of insulin, reduce utilization of glucose in adipose tissue and muscle.
- Insulin concentrations rise after a meal so that postprandial insulin can orchestrate the distribution of energy from food (see **19**).
  - ◇ During fasting insulin levels are low, but after eating insulin secretion rapidly increases in healthy subjects.

The structure of insulin

◆ Insulin is a peptide hormone, with 51 amino acids arranged in two chains linked by two disulfide bonds.

◇ Some of these amino acids are different in patients with diabetes associated with mutant insulins, others are different in other mammalian species (cattle, pigs), while others have been modified in therapeutic insulin analogs (e.g. Lantus, Humalog).

◆ In the synthesis of insulin, translation of mRNA yields preproinsulin, a prohormone containing 110 amino acids, which undergoes post-translational modification prior to the release of the mature insulin molecule.

◇ Removal of 24 amino acids from preproinsulin yields proinsulin, with 86 amino acids, which is then stored in secretory granules within the β cell.

◇ In healthy subjects, over 90% of proinsulin is converted to mature insulin by the removal of the metabolically inert C-peptide component (**23**).

◆ C-peptide is only partially extracted by the liver, so levels of this protein can be used as an index of insulin secretion. In healthy subjects only small amounts (<10% of mature insulin output) of proinsulin and partially split proinsulin are released.

◇ These ratios are characteristically disturbed in certain pathological states, including autonomous insulin secretion from an insulinoma and in type 2 diabetes, and will be low or undetectable in cases of surreptitious administration of exogenous insulin.

◇ Assay of these substances may therefore, in some circumstances, prove helpful in the differential diagnosis of hypoglycemia.

◇ Proinsulin may accumulate in renal failure and is elevated in familial hyperproinsulinemia.

◆ Substances stimulating the synthesis and storage of insulin include glucose, mannose, leucine, arginine, hormones such as GLP-1, and a variety of metabolizable sugars or sugar derivatives. Most of these also promote secretion and these factors are collectively termed secretagogues.

23 Structure of insulin and proinsulin. Proinsulin synthesized in the pancreatic β cells is converted to insulin by the removal of the 31 amino acids that form the C-peptide protein in the center of the sequence; the two other ends (the B chain and A chain) remain connected by disulfide bonds.

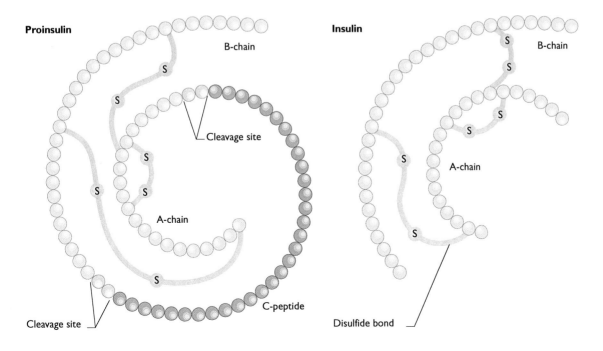

Proinsulin

B-chain

Cleavage site

A-chain

Cleavage site

C-peptide

Insulin

B-chain

A-chain

Disulfide bond

Normal insulin secretion and kinetics

- The mechanisms regulating insulin release are the focus of much research.
- It is known that there is an ATP-dependent, sulfonylurea-sensitive potassium (K^+) channel whose closure is a late event in the intracellular signaling mechanism within the β cell. Potassium channel closure triggers calcium influx and exocytosis (**24**).
- A wide range of secretagogues will stimulate closure of the K^+ channel. The most important of these stimulants is hyperglycemia.
    - ◇ Other secretagogues include mannose, lactate, some amino acids, glucagon, glucose-dependent insulinotrophic peptide (GIP), cholecystokinin, vasoactive intestinal peptide (VIP), ghrelin, glucagon-like peptide-1 (GLP-1), sulfonylureas, and parasympathetic cholinergic (muscarinic) nerve activity; many have synergistic effects.

- Conversely, insulin secretion is inhibited by both neural sympathetic tone and circulating catecholamines.
- A combination of cephalic and gastric effects makes oral glucose a more potent stimulus to insulin secretion than an equivalent amount of intravenous glucose. This is known as the 'incretin' effect and is, at least in part, attributable to gut-derived hormones such as GIP and GLP-1.
- In healthy adults, insulin is secreted in pulses with a periodicity of 11–15 min.
    - ◇ Stimuli of insulin secretion increase the frequency and amplitude of these pulses.
    - ◇ Approximately 30–40 units (240 pmol) of insulin are secreted every 24 hours in healthy subjects of normal weight.
    - ◇ Insulin secretion is basal (0.25–1.0 U/h) when glycemia is below a threshold level of about 5 mmol/l (90 mg/dl) and insulin output is maximal at glycemia of 15–20 mmol/l (270–360 mg/dl).
- Insulin is secreted into the portal venous system and must traverse the liver prior to reaching the systemic circulation.
    - ◇ The liver is thus exposed to insulin concentrations approximately three times higher than other tissues when insulin is secreted endogenously.
    - ◇ About 50% of secreted insulin is extracted and degraded in the 'first pass' through the liver; much of the residue is broken down by the kidneys.
- The pulsatile pattern of insulin secretion and clearance is controlled not only by prevailing blood glucose concentration, but also by the secretagogues mentioned above.
    - ◇ It is not hard to appreciate the difficulty in replicating such a physiological appearance of insulin with the subcutaneous administration of exogenous insulin.

24 **Insulin secretion.** Extracellular glucose is transported into the β cell via the GLUT2 receptor, where it is converted into glucose-6-phosphate by the enzyme glucokinase (1). Glycolysis within the mitochondrion generates ATP, which leads to the closure of ATP-sensitive potassium channels (2) and depolarization of the cell membrane (3). This opens the voltage-dependent calcium channels (4) and allows the influx of calcium and the subsequent release of insulin (5).

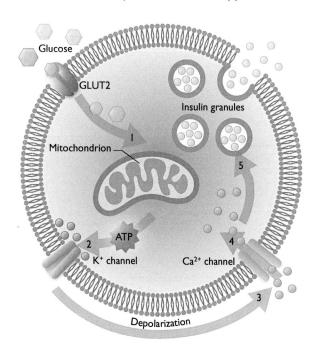

Hyperglycemia is the most important stimulant for secretion of insulin.

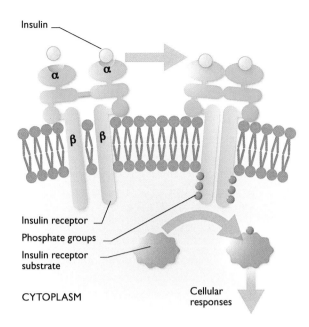

25 Insulin receptor action. When insulin binds to the two extracellular α subunits of the receptor, the transmembrane β subunits transmit a signal that activates their protein kinase domain. Phosphorylation of the insulin receptor substrate triggers further reactions, leading to the uptake of glucose.

◆ Autocrine and paracrine regulation of insulin secretion by pancreatic and gut hormones (which may reach very high concentrations within the islet) are incompletely understood. Increased secretion of insulin involves recruitment of more β cells to the secreting mode.

◆ Fasting peripheral insulin concentrations vary between 3 and 15 mU/l (~20–100 pmol/l), as measured by radio immunoassays in healthy subjects, the higher values being associated with increasing age and obesity.
  ◇ After a typical mixed meal (700–800 kcal), the peak plasma insulin concentration will be 40–80 mU/l (~280–560 pmol/l) in young, lean adults.

◆ The half-life of insulin injected into a peripheral vein is 2–6 minutes, with the liver clearing most of this insulin and smaller amounts being cleared in other tissues having insulin receptors, such as skeletal muscle, although there is also nonreceptor-mediated clearance by a variety of tissue proteases.

The insulin receptor

◆ Insulin's main glucoregulatory effects are mediated by the insulin receptor – a transmembrane receptor coded by chromosome 19 and found on insulin-sensitive cells. This receptor is a glycoprotein, comprising four peptide subchains, two α and two β subunits, linked by disulfide bridges.

◆ There are two receptor isoforms, IR-A and IR-D, formed by alternate splicing.

◆ The DNA sequence and amino acid structure of the insulin receptor show homology with those of the insulin-like growth factor-1 (IGF-1) receptor.

◆ When insulin binds to the extracellular domain of the α subunit of the insulin receptor, an enzyme (tyrosine kinase) on the the intracellular domain of the β subunit is activated; the signal is thus transferred across the membrane. Activation of other intracellular enzymes follows (**25**).

◆ After activation, the insulin–receptor complex is internalized by endocytosis. The receptor is later recycled to the cell surface. Internalization of the insulin receptor is important (and possibly essential) for insulin signals to reach the nucleus and influence cell growth and protein synthesis. Internalization is also a route by which insulin is cleared from the circulation and degraded.

◆ Rare DNA mutations of the insulin receptor have been identified:
  ◇ Leprechaunism and Rabson–Mendenhall syndrome result in severe glucose intolerance with resistance to exogenous insulin and profoundly disordered growth, unlike the 'typical' insulin resistance. These mutations are usually lethal in infancy and adolescence, respectively.

◆ There are also commoner, 'milder' polymorphisms of the insulin receptor gene, but these appear to explain only a small proportion of the marked variance in population insulin sensitivity and are considered a rare (<5%) cause of type 2 diabetes.
  ◇ Most recognized insulin receptor gene mutations are not sufficient alone to cause diabetes, but render it more common in the presence of other risk factors.

The actions of insulin

◆ Insulin has widespread actions, both inhibitory and stimulatory (**26**, **27**).

◇ The mechanisms of the glucoregulatory action of insulin have been the subject of extensive research. These glucoregulatory and antilipolytic effects of insulin are rapid, occurring within a few minutes.

◇ Insulin has effects on growth regulation and catabolism (synthesis of new proteins) which occur over hours or days. Much less is known about the other possible actions, including effects on blood vessels (vascular smooth muscle proliferation, vasodilatation), the central nervous system (CNS) (appetite, learning, memory), and the immune response (apoptosis and anti-inflammation).

◆ There are individual dose–response curves for the different actions of insulin in different tissues. For example:

◇ *Antilipolytic action in adipose tissue:* the ED_{50} (the effective dose or concentration of insulin that produces 50% of the maximal effect) is <20 mU/l (~140 pmol/l) (and for some adipose depots <70 pmol/l).

◇ *Inhibition of hepatic glucose output (HGO):* ED_{50} of 30–50 mU/l (~210–350 pmol/l).

◇ *Stimulation of glucose uptake into skeletal muscle:* ED_{50} of 50–70 mU/l (~350–490 pmol/l).

◇ A doubling of insulin concentration inhibits hepatic glucose output by around 80% and increases peripheral glucose utilization by around 20%.

◆ These differential effects on lipolysis, HGO, and glucose uptake are probably responsible for the fact that most individuals with type 2 diabetes retain sufficient insulin action to avoid the development of ketoacidosis (for many years), despite the clear defect in glucoregulation.

26 Actions of insulin. As well as promoting the uptake of glucose and inhibiting gluconeogenesis, insulin is significant in the metabolism of lipids, promoting synthesis of free fatty acids in the liver and inhibiting the breakdown of fats in adipose tissues. The insulin receptor facilitates uptake of amino acids and glucose across the cell membrane and activates protein, glycogen, and triglyceride synthesis.

Insulin is significant in carbohydrate, protein, and lipid metabolism.

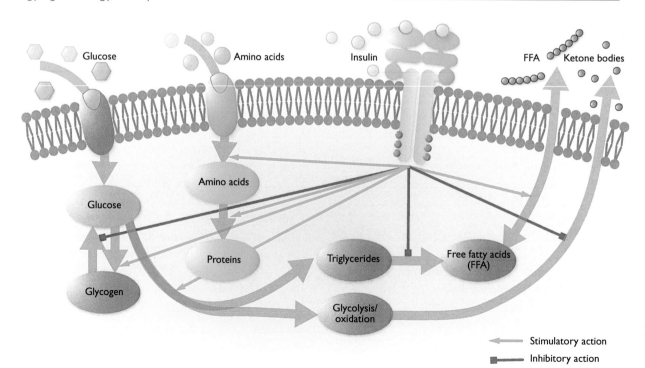

Actions of insulin

TISSUES	ACTIONS	SUGGESTED MECHANISM
Liver	Inhibition of hepatic glucose output	Limitation of substrate supply
	Stimulation of hepatic glycogen storage	Inhibition of glycogenolysis
	Stimulation of hepatic glycolysis for intermediary metabolism	Inhibition of gluconeogenesis; stimulation of glycogen synthase
	Stimulation of hepatic lipogenesis	Stimulation of phosphofructokinase
	Stimulation of hepatic glucose oxidation	Stimulation of pyruvate dehydrogenase
Skeletal muscle	Stimulation of glucose transport	Activation of glucose transporter (GLUT4)
	Stimulation of muscle glycogen synthesis	Stimulation of glycogen synthase
	Stimulation of muscle glycolysis	Stimulation of phosphofructokinase
Adipose tissue	Inhibition of lipolysis (stored lipid)	Inhibition of hormone sensitive lipase
	Promotion of re-esterification	Increased supply of glycerol 3-phosphate
	Stimulation of lipolysis (circulating lipid)	Stimulation of lipoprotein lipase
	Increased glucose uptake	Several (probably as for muscle/liver)
Central nervous system	Satiety	Uncertain
	Changes in sympathetic tone	Uncertain
	Postprandial thermogenesis	Uncertain
Other	Promotes DNA synthesis	Uncertain
	Promotes RNA synthesis	Various
	Stimulation of amino acid uptake	Uncertain
	Na^+, K^+-ATPase stimulation	Increase in intracellular energy availability
	Na^+/H^+ antiport activation	Uncertain
	Na^+ retention	Probably several mechanisms

27 Actions of insulin. Insulin affects virtually every tissue in the body.

- The different actions of insulin have different time courses:
  - ◇ Glucoregulatory and antilipolytic actions occur within a few minutes, while growth regulation and synthesis of new proteins occur over periods of hours or days.
- ◇ Intravenous injection of insulin typically has little effect on blood glucose for 2–5 minutes; the maximal hypoglycemic action occurs after 5–15 minutes.
- ◇ Insulin stimulation of skeletal muscle glucose uptake declines with a half-life of 10–20 minutes after the insulin stimulus is removed.

◆ Proinsulin and partially split proinsulin have metabolic activity generally similar to that of insulin, although plasma half-life is three to five times longer and biological potency is only 8–15% that of insulin. Proinsulin may be relatively more potent in terms of hepatic activity and less potent in terms of peripheral glucose uptake.

◇ In sum, proinsulin has a limited role in general peripheral glucose metabolism but may have a relatively more important role in hepatic metabolism.

Second messenger systems

◆ Insulin can have multiple actions even on a single responsive cell and hence there are several different intracellular pathways mediating these actions (see **26**).

◇ Glucoregulatory and antilipolytic responses are rapid and probably mediated via serine and threonine kinases and cyclic adenosine monophosphate (cAMP).

◇ Stimulation of lipid and protein synthesis, inhibition of proteolysis, the nuclear transcription of RNA, and the replication of DNA are slower and act via different second messenger systems.

◇ As a result of these second messenger cascades, GLUT proteins are translocated to the surface membrane of the cell and increase glucose flux into the cytoplasm.

◆ The actions of insulin in stimulating DNA transcription and mRNA translation do not depend upon the insulin receptor kinase activity and second messenger systems discussed above, nor on the IGF receptors described below, but involve direct effects within the nucleus and ribosome.

Insulin-like growth factors (IGFs)

◆ In addition to its acute effects on glucose uptake and release and on lipid metabolism, insulin has growth-promoting activity in a variety of tissue-culture models.

◇ Two protein hormones, IGF-1 and IGF-2, have actions that partially resemble these actions of insulin. The amino acid sequences of these proteins and the base sequences of their coding DNA are known and show homology with those of insulin.

◆ IGFs are weak agonists for the insulin receptor and have weak glucoregulatory and antilipolytic effects. In addition, they have growth-promoting effects mediated by two IGF receptors.

◆ Insulin is a weak agonist of IGF receptors.

Abnormalities of insulin synthesis and secretion

◆ The most common abnormality is the progressive loss of normal pulsatility, delayed insulin response to hyperglycemia, and gradual loss of insulin secretory capacity seen as obese individuals move towards type 2 diabetes. The progressive loss of insulin secretion in type 1 diabetes has a different natural history.

◆ However, there are also some rarer, genetic abnormalities of insulin structure involving mutations of the DNA code for insulin and hence altered amino acid sequences. Consequences include the inability to cleave insulin from proinsulin, and impaired receptor binding.

◇ For these variants, there is reduced biological activity of the secretory product. This gives a propensity to diabetes, although individuals who can sustain a compensatory hypersecretion may avoid it.

◆ There are also recognized polymorphisms that affect the insulin secretory mechanism (e.g. calpain 10, a molecule that promotes the fusion of the secretory granule with the cell membrane) and are associated with diabetes.

CHAPTER 3

Type 1 diabetes

Epidemiology

- Type 1 diabetes is the result of severe insulin deficiency leading to insulin-dependent diabetes. It is one of the most common chronic diseases of childhood.
- Highest incidence rates of type 1A (autoimmune) diabetes are in Finland and the island of Sardinia. The frequency of type 1A diabetes in Europe is comparatively high compared with the rest of the world, higher in temperate zones and developed countries, correlating with gross national product as an index of wealth.
- Type 1B (idiopathic) diabetes has been noted in Japanese patients, who progress rapidly to insulin dependence in adult life without diabetes-associated antibodies but with increased serum amylase consistent with a subacute pancreatitis.
- The incidence of type 1 diabetes is increasing (**28**), particularly in children under the age of 5 years. The peak incidence is reached around the time of puberty, but it can present at any age.
  - ◇ In a multicenter study, based on 2002–2003 data, 15,000 young people in the USA were newly diagnosed with type 1 diabetes annually. Non-Hispanic white youth had the highest rate of new cases (**29**).

Type 1 diabetes can present at any age.

---

29 Diabetes in the young. The average rate of new cases of diabetes (2002–2003) among under-20s in the USA was 19 per 100,000 each year for type 1 diabetes and 5.3 per 100,000 for type 2 diabetes.

Worldwide type 1 diabetes incidence in children (2007)

Children 0–14 years (billions)	1.8
Children with type 1 diabetes	440,000
Type 1 diabetes prevalence (per 100,000)	24
Annual increase of incidence (%)	3.0
Newly-diagnosed cases/year (estimated)	70,000

28 Incidence of childhood type 1 diabetes. There is enormous variation in the incidence of type 1 diabetes, from 0.1/100,000 per year in China and Venezuela to 36.8/100,000 per year in Sardinia and 36.5/100,000 per year in Finland. Results from 37 studies in 27 countries during 1960 to 1996 showed that the overall annual increase in incidence was around 3.0%. Some 70,000 children worldwide are expected to develop type 1 diabetes each year.

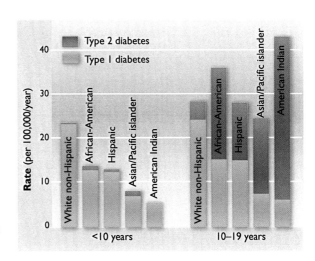

Diagnostic differences between LADA, KPD, and double diabetes

	AGE	WEIGHT LOSS	KETOSIS	INSULIN SECRETION	HLA RISK	DIABETES-SPECFIC AUTOANTIBODIES
LADA	Adult	Absent	Absent	Present/declines	Present	Present
KPD	Young/adult	Present	Present	Variable	In some	In some
Double diabetes	Young	Absent	Absent	Present	To be studied	Present

◆ Slow progression to insulin deficiency occurs in about 10% of adult patients who present initially with noninsulin-dependent diabetes. This is often called latent autoimmune diabetes of adults (LADA).

◇ LADA is characterized by the presence of diabetes-associated antibodies, including glutamic acid decarboxylase antibody (GADA). However, some patients appear to have features of both type 1 and type 2 diabetes (called double-diabetes) and some ethnic groups, including those of Hispanic or African origin, may present with ketoacidosis which later passes through a period of not requiring insulin treatment, so-called ketosis-prone diabetes (KPD) (**30**).

30 Type I diabetes subtypes seen in adulthood. The differential characteristics of these forms of diabetes overlap in part, reflecting their complex and diverse pathogenesis.

◆ The striking discordance between identical twins must be due to nongenetic, probably environmental factors. These environmental factors probably operate in early life, even *in utero*, at least in those cases which present in childhood. Patients presenting in adulthood have a more potent environmental input but the origins of that effect are unclear. The nature of the environmental factor or factors is also unknown but candidates include viruses and food, such as early exposure to cow's milk.

Causes of type I diabetes

◆ Type 1 diabetes is an immune-mediated organ-specific disease. The disease is induced by an environmental event or events operating in a genetically susceptible individual (**31**).

◆ Many genes are implicated in the genetic susceptibility to type 1 diabetes; the most important are in the histocompatibility leukocyte antigen (HLA) region of chromosome 6.

◆ The risk of developing childhood-onset type 1 diabetes is about 1:400 in the general population but 1:2 in an identical twin of a young diabetic twin, 1:10 in the identical twin of an adult diabetic twin, and 1:17 in a sibling of a subject with type 1 diabetes; the risk is only 1:5 if the sibling is HLA-identical to the affected sibling.

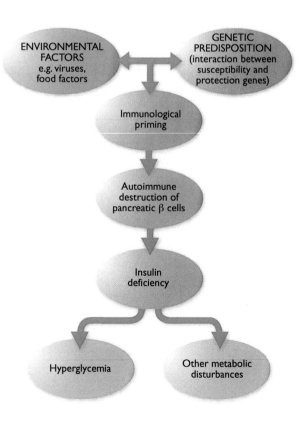

31 Etiological events. Type I diabetes is an immune-mediated disease, induced by environmental determinants in a genetically susceptible individual.

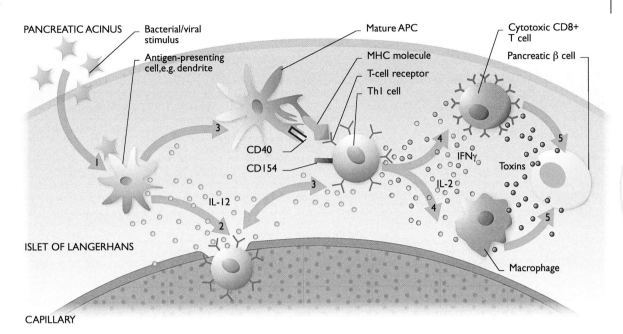

PANCREATIC ACINUS — Bacterial/viral stimulus

Antigen-presenting cell, e.g. dendrite

Mature APC

MHC molecule

T-cell receptor

Th1 cell

Cytotoxic CD8+ T cell

Pancreatic β cell

CD40

CD154

IL-12

IFNγ

IL-2

Toxins

ISLET OF LANGERHANS

Macrophage

CAPILLARY

10% of patients presenting with adult-onset diabetes have autoimmune diabetes.

- The risk of developing diabetes by age 20 years is greater with a type 1 diabetic father (8%) than with a type 1 diabetic mother (2%); this discrepancy may be a result of imprinted maternal genes or because fetal exposure to maternal GADAs may be protective to the offspring.
- Whatever the nature of the environmental effect, the interaction of environmental and genetic factors at different stages leads to induction of immune changes, including activation of T lymphocytes and B lymphocytes, with the latter producing autoantibodies.
  - ◇ The destructive immune response targets the pancreatic islets, specifically the insulin-secreting cells, with complete or partial destruction of them.
  - ◇ The destruction can be mediated directly by cellular processes or indirectly through the release of cytokines and chemokines (**32**). At diagnosis, children show lymphocytes and macrophages surrounding and infiltrating the islets (**33**).
  - ◇ The younger the onset of the disease, the more severe is this destructive immune process.

32 Immune-mediated destruction of pancreatic β cells. Upon activation (1), antigen-presenting cells (APCs), such as dendritic cells, produce IL-12 cytokines that stimulate the production of Th1 lymphocytes (2). T-cell receptor (TCR) and CD154 molecules on the surface of the Th1 cell bind to the MHC and CD40 molecules on the surface of the APC (3). Th1 lymphocytes also produce large amounts of interferon-gamma (IFN-γ) which, together with IL-2 cytokines, induces macrophages to become cytotoxic, and also stimulates cytotoxic CD8+ cells (4). Both of these release mediators that are toxic to pancreatic islet cells (5).

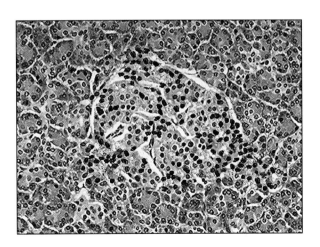

33 Insulitis. Lymphocytic infiltration in a pancreatic islet, suggesting an altered immune response.

Prediction of type 1 diabetes

- The immune changes associated with type 1 diabetes can be detected months, or even years, before the clinical onset of the disease. These changes, notably the presence of autoantibodies, can predict the disease, with some antibodies and particularly combinations of antibodies being more predictive than others (**34**).
  - ◇ The ability to predict the disease raises the hope that we may eventually be able to prevent it and clinical trials are now under way.
- Autoimmune diseases show three features:
  - ◇ Defined autoantigens and autoantibodies must be present.
  - ◇ Passive transfer of T lymphocytes (specific or nonspecific) must lead to disease development.
  - ◇ Immunomodulation of subjects with disease must ameliorate symptoms.
- The first of these is true for type 1 diabetes and the autoantibodies to autoantigens can predict the disease with a degree of certainty. Some immunomodulation therapies can modify, albeit transiently, the disease process.
- Type 1 diabetes is associated with other autoimmune diseases, including Hashimoto's thyroiditis, adrenalitis, celiac disease and pernicious anemia (with vitamin B12 deficiency).

The presence of autoantibodies before clinical onset can predict diabetes.

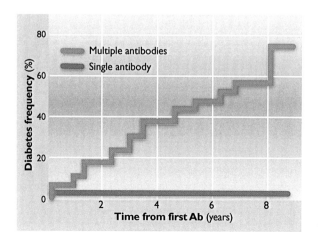

Genetic factors

- Type 1 diabetes is genetically determined as evidenced by family, twin, and genetic studies. Type 1 diabetes is more frequent in siblings of diabetic patients (e.g. in the UK, 6% by age 30 versus the expected 0.4% by age 30). Higher concordance rates in identical compared with nonidentical twins is consistent with a genetic influence in type 1 diabetes. About 40% of identical twins with type 1 diabetes have a co-twin with the disease (i.e. they are concordant for type 1 diabetes), though that proportion falls as the age at diagnosis of the index twin rises.
  - ◇ The remarkably low twin concordance rate for adult-onset type 1 diabetes implies a limited genetic impact, much less than in childhood-onset disease.
- HLA genes are associated with an increased risk of a number of autoimmune diseases. Genes encoding these HLA molecules are found within the major histocompatibility complex (MHC) on the short arm of chromosome 6 (**35**). HLA genes are highly polymorphic and this region has been in balanced polymorphism for at least 10 million years. HLA associations with type 1 diabetes probably operate through susceptibility to undefined infections.
  - ◇ This MHC complex is a polymorphic gene complex with multiple alleles at each genetic locus. The MHC is divided into class I (HLA -A, -B, and -C), class II (HLA-DR, -DQ, and -DP), and class III (genes for complement components).
  - ◇ The class I and class II proteins are transmembrane cell surface glycoproteins involved in both self and foreign antigen presentation to T lymphocytes.

34 Islet autoimmunity. The German BABYDIAB study monitored 1610 newborn children, who had at least 1 parent with type 1 diabetes, for islet autoantibody and diabetes development. Over a period of 11 years, 51 children developed multiple islet autoantibodies, of whom 23 developed the disease. The cumulative risk for developing diabetes within 5 years after first becoming autoantibody positive was 40% in offspring who had multiple autoantibodies and 3% in those who had single autoantibodies.

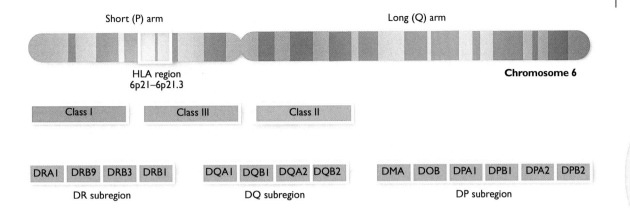

HLA region
6p21–6p21.3

Chromosome 6

| Class I | | Class III | | Class II | |

| DRA1 | DRB9 | DRB3 | DRB1 | DQA1 | DQB1 | DQA2 | DQB2 | DMA | DOB | DPA1 | DPB1 | DPA2 | DPB2 |

DR subregion   DQ subregion   DP subregion

35 Genetic factors. There are numerous regions of the genome associated with type 1 diabetes risk, with IDDM1 on chromosome 6 being the most important. HLA genes within this region account for almost 50% of genetic susceptibility to type 1 diabetes.

◆ Class II genes are more important than Class I genes, and DQ genes are more important than DR genes.
  ◇ About 95% of European patients have either HLA-DR3 or HLA-DR4, compared with about 60% of the general population, and specific alleles of HLA-DR3 and HLA-DR4 have been identified that are associated with diabetes susceptibility.
  ◇ Other alleles are associated with disease protection, e.g. one haplotype (HLA-DR2, DQB1*0602) is found in about 20% of some populations, but in less than 1% of those that develop the disease.
  ◇ The heterozygous alleles associated with disease susceptibility, HLA-DR3, DQB1*0201 and HLA-DR4, DQB1*0302, decline in frequency with age at diagnosis, while, in adult-onset diabetes, the protective HLA haplotype carries less protection.
◆ In the HLA molecule, individual residues (i.e. specific amino acids at certain positions) confer a particular susceptibility or protection from disease.

There are 40 genetic variants associated with type 1 diabetes.

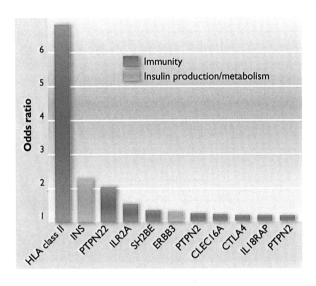

36 Selected genes associated with type 1 diabetes.
More than 40 genetic loci that underlie susceptibility to type 1 diabetes have now been identified. While the HLA gene is the most significant, others such as INS, which regulates insulin production and CTLA4, the cytotoxic T-lymphocyte antigen gene, are also of great interest. The graph indicates the estimated odds ratio for risk alleles at each of the indicated loci. *Adapted from Todd et al.*

◆ Other gene polymorphisms are associated with type 1 diabetes, including a gene within the insulin gene upstream promoter region.
  ◇ Of particular note, the IFIH1 gene plays a role in anti-viral defense, clearly implicating viruses in the pathogenesis of the disease.
◆ In total, there are some 40 genetic variants associated with type 1 diabetes but only 10 are known to have a function, such as genes involved in T cell immune responses (**36**).

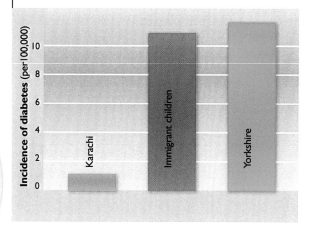

37 Nongenetic factors. The incidence of type 1 diabetes amongst Pakistani immigrants to Yorkshire between 1978 and 1990 showed an increase to levels comparable with those of the local population. *Adapted from Staines & Bodansky, 1997.*

Nongenetic factors

◆ Nongenetic factors are important in causing type 1 diabetes, as shown by studies of populations, twins, and migrant populations.

◇ Population studies reveal changes in disease incidence within a genetically stable population, both in populations that do not move and those that do.

◇ There has been a striking increase in the incidence of type 1 diabetes in children diagnosed under 5 years of age in Europe within a generation, implicating nongenetic factors.

◇ An increase has been reported in migrating populations, e.g. Asian children who migrated to Britain from Karachi showed an increased disease risk from 3.1/100,000 per year in 1978–81 to 11.7/100,000 per year in 1988–90, much higher than in their native Karachi (1/100,000 per year) (**37**).

◇ Such increases in disease risk in young children could be due to an accelerated progression to disease, or to an increased disease risk, or both. Current evidence supports both factors being involved.

38 Disease progression. Time-related decline in β-cell mass, showing critical transitions from genetic susceptibility to frank diabetes. *Adapted from Eisenbarth, 1986.*

◆ A range of environmental factors may cause autoimmune diseases. These factors include:

◇ Increased hygiene and decreased rates of infection.

◇ Temperate climate.

◇ Vaccinations and antibiotics.

◇ Increasing wealth (possibly all relevant for most autoimmune and atopic diseases).

◆ For type 1 diabetes, other factors are:

◇ Overcrowding in childhood and virus infections.

◇ Reduced rates or duration of breast feeding.

◇ Early exposure to cow's milk.

◇ Reduced vitamin D consumption.

◆ Several or one of these factors could account for the disease in any given individual.

Development of type 1 diabetes

Pancreatic β-cell dysfunction

◆ There is a continuous spectrum of loss of insulin secretory capacity associated with autoimmune diabetes. The severity of the destructive immune effect is age-related, being more severe in children than in adults and more severe in adults with type 1 diabetes than in adults with LADA.

◆ Some individuals, before they develop type 1 diabetes, pass through a 'prediabetic' stage of impaired glucose tolerance or even noninsulin-requiring diabetes, before becoming frankly insulin-dependent (**38**).

◆ The rate of progression to clinical diabetes is more rapid in those patients presenting at less than 5 years of age than in patients presenting with diabetes much later in life.

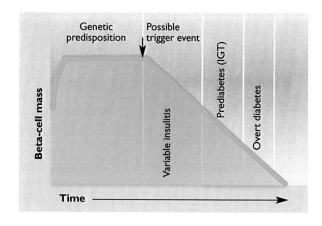

Insulin resistance

◆ The normal relationship between insulin sensitivity relative to insulin secretion is disrupted in the 'prediabetic' phase, just as it is in type 2 diabetes.

◆ Those autoantibody-positive individuals who develop type 1 diabetes show changes in insulin sensitivity during this period. It follows that metabolic decompensation, which leads to frank diabetes, can result from any cause of reduced insulin sensitivity, as is seen with increased linear growth and increased childhood obesity, both of which are related to age at presentation.

Mortality

◆ The Pittsburgh Epidemiology of Diabetes Complications study has demonstrated that the pattern of causes of death changes, depending on the duration of type 1 diabetes (**39**).

◇ Cardiovascular disease was the principal cause of death among people who had had type 1 diabetes for more than 30 years.

◇ Renal disease formed the largest proportion of causes of death among people whose disease duration was between 10 and 19 years.

◇ In contrast, for those who died less than 10 years after diagnosis, the major causes of death were other diabetes-related complications such as hypoglycemia and diabetic ketoacidosis.

◆ Recent studies also identify acute complications of diabetes as the major cause of death in teenagers and cardiovascular disease as the major cause of death in people over 30 years of age. It has also been noted that South Asian patients with insulin-treated diabetes suffer an exceptionally high mortality, which may be related to a higher risk of cardiovascular disease.

◆ Cancer mortality among people with type 1 diabetes is thought to be generally similar to that of the general population.

◇ There may be greater incidence of ovarian cancer and mortality, as implied by at least one study.

◇ Recent papers have questioned whether the use of an insulin analog, glargine insulin, could be associated with an excess risk of breast cancer, but this observation requires confirmation in larger, prospective studies and the current recommendation is that clinicians should be cautious but continue use of this therapy, much as before.

39 Diabetes complications. The Pittsburgh EDC study followed five cohorts of participants over a 30-year period, with renal failure and coronary artery disease (as well as mortality, proliferative retinopathy, and neuropathy) status assessed at 20, 25, and 30 years. There was a decreasing trend for renal failure, but less so for CAD.

Cardiovascular disease is the major cause of death in patients who have had type 1 diabetes for over 30 years.

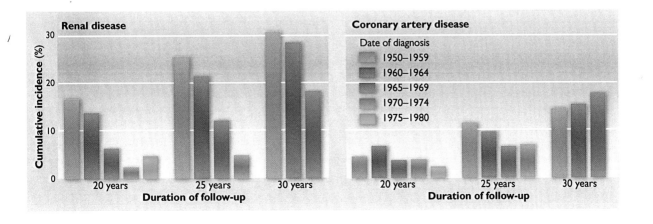

Screening for potential type I diabetes

- Autoimmune diseases are the third leading cause of morbidity and mortality in the developed world, surpassed only by cancer and heart disease.
- Autoimmune diseases are complex, chronic disorders that develop over the course of years and are characterized by autoantibodies, which appear in the peripheral blood months, even years, before the onset of clinical symptoms. Since the genes associated with autoimmune diseases are susceptibility genes, and therefore carry a limited predictive value, attention has turned to the immune response, and specifically disease-associated autoantibodies, as potential predictors.
- Screening for autoantibodies as predictors of disease has been convincingly demonstrated for a number of autoimmune diseases, including type 1 diabetes. These studies, involving thousands of subjects, showed that autoantibodies:
  - ◇ Can appear at an early age, even around the time of birth.
  - ◇ Can precede the clinical onset of diabetes by some years.
  - ◇ Recognize different autoantigens and some antigen-specific autoantibodies are more predictive of type 1 diabetes than others (e.g. autoantibodies recognizing glutamic acid decarboxylase [GAD] are less predictive than those recognizing insulinoma-associated antigen-2 [IA-2], zinc transporter 8 [ZnT8] or insulin [IAA]).
  - ◇ Have a positive predictive value that increases for one, two, or three autoantibodies from approximately 10% to 50% and 80%, respectively, within 5 years and even higher thereafter.
- The success of screening with autoantibodies for type 1 diabetes suggests that autoantibody screening will be useful in predicting other chronic autoimmune diseases. Such screening could be used to identify subjects at risk in the immediate family or general population, in order to identify those suitable for prevention therapy when it becomes available. They can also be used to classify the disease, notably when patients present with noninsulin-dependent diabetes as adults, of whom some 5–10% have autoimmune type 1 diabetes.

CHAPTER 4

Type 2 diabetes

Epidemiology

◆ Type 2 diabetes is a common chronic disease of global importance (see p. 12). Most patients (>85%) with diabetes have type 2 diabetes.

◆ The rate of increase of type 2 diabetes is such that there is effectively a global epidemic of it. The WHO estimated that 30 million people had diabetes in 1985; in 2011 the estimate was 366 million, and projections are that numbers will reach 552 million by 2030.

◆ Diabetes has traditionally been viewed as a disease of rich countries. However, recent estimates of diabetes prevalence show that 80% of people with diabetes live in countries classified by the World Bank as low- and middle-income countries, and this proportion is set to increase.

◆ The prevalence of type 2 diabetes is related to increasing age, increasing calorie intake, increasing obesity (**40**) and reduced physical activity. Pregnancy, certain drug therapy, and intercurrent illness are all associated with precipitating diabetes.

◆ Type 2 diabetes can remain undiagnosed for many years.

◆ Using the WHO criteria, the prevalence of known diabetes in the UK is about 20% and in members of affected families about 30%.

◇ However, in some previously undeveloped societies, recently exposed to the Western lifestyle, such as Pima Indians in the United States and the Naruans from Micronesia, the prevalence is up to 70%.

◆ Recognized morphological associations of type 2 diabetes include shorter stature (by 1–4 cm compared to nondiabetic subjects) with obesity of the 'android' (also known as 'apple', 'upper body', 'central' or 'visceral') type, marked by a high waist:hip ratio, low capillary density in skeletal muscle, with high ratios of slow twitch: fast twitch muscle fibers.

40 Obesity in developed countries. Levels of obesity have been increasing consistently over the past three decades (*OECD data 1996–2003*).

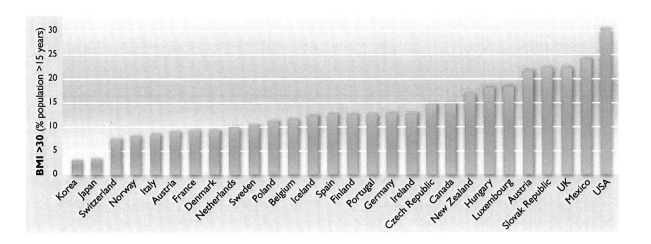

Causes of type 2 diabetes

- Type 2 diabetes is probably not a single condition. Some late-onset diabetes, initially presumed to be type 2, will turn out to be latent autoimmune diabetes in adults (LADA), while other patients thought to have type 2 diabetes may upon investigation be shown to have secondary types such as pancreatic.
- In all patients with type 2 diabetes, there is both insulin resistance and relative insulin deficiency.
- With time (typically 5–15 years from diagnosis), glycemic control in type 2 patients usually becomes more difficult, insulin deficiency more apparent and a subgroup of patients will become ketosis-prone. Data from the UKPDS trial suggested that the average time to insulin use was approximately 8 years after diagnosis of type 2 diabetes and confirmed the clinical impression of a progressive rather than static disease process.

Determinants and risk factors for type 2 diabetes

Lifestyle and behavior related	'Westernization, urbanization, modernization' Obesity (including distribution of obesity and duration) Physical inactivity Diet Stress
Genetic	Genetic markers 'Thrifty gene(s)' Family history
Demographic	Sex, age, ethnicity Other demographic characteristics
Metabolic determinants and intermediate risk categories	Impaired glucose tolerance Insulin resistance Pregnancy-related determinants (parity, gestational diabetes, diabetes in offspring of women with diabetes during pregnancy, intrauterine mal- or overnutrition)

41 **Risk factors.** The main determinants for type 2 diabetes are linked to social factors, such as socio-economic status. Age, family history, poor diet and physical inactivity are the main risk factors.

Type 2 diabetes is associated with both insulin resistance and relative insulin deficiency.

Environmental risk factors

- The typical patient with type 2 diabetes is overweight (average body mass index [BMI] at presentation, >27 kg/m^2), with a central distribution of obesity (most conveniently assessed by waist circumference, or waist:hip ratio) conferring risk which is independent of, and additional to, that of elevated BMI (**41**).
- Other independent risk factors for type 2 diabetes include lack of exercise, being born to a mother with gestational diabetes , being of exceptionally high or low birth weight.
  - ◇ Low birth weight is postulated by the 'Barker Hypothesis' to predispose to diabetes and obesity by various mechanisms, including switching on 'thrifty' genes to counter the effects of intrauterine malnutrition.
- Leaner patients with type 2 diabetes tend to show more severe insulin deficiency (and within this subgroup one typically finds LADA patients).
- Greater degrees of obesity are associated with more insulin resistance.
- There is longstanding controversy as to whether, for the type 2 diabetes typical of patients of European origin, the prime defect in glucose homoeostasis is insulin deficiency or insulin resistance, or both. Given that many individuals with severe insulin resistance do not have diabetes and that some patients with type 2 diabetes have little insulin resistance, it is probable that insulin resistance alone is not the cause; rather, some degree of β-cell dysfunction (either as an inherited tendency or a result of reduced β-cell function as part of a degenerative process) is the *sine qua non* of type 2 diabetes.
  - ◇ Such β-cell dysfunction may take the form of a *relative* lack of insulin secretion and/or of abnormal patterns of insulin secretion.
  - ◇ Such abnormalities have been described in patients who later developed type 2 diabetes and include changes in the amplitude and frequency of insulin secretory pulses, and in the loss of first-phase insulin secretion with prolongation and augmentation of second-phase secretion.

◇ These abnormalities of insulin secretion have been shown to be largely reversible after certain forms of bariatric surgery for morbid obesity in patients with type 2 diabetes.

◆ Population studies indicate that the concurrent existence in an individual of both a cause for insulin resistance (usually obesity) and of a relatively low insulin secretory reserve predicts the onset of type 2 diabetes.

◆ The differentiation of type 2 diabetes and 'secondary' diabetes can be difficult.

◇ 'Secondary diabetes' implies that another disease process has caused or substantially contributed to the diabetes (see p. 16). While there is good understanding of the natural history and treatment approach for type 2 diabetes, this is less so for secondary diabetes. Occasionally, the secondary diabetes may be significantly improved by treating the primary condition.

Genetic factors

◆ Family studies suggest that type 2 diabetes is strongly inheritable:

◇ Concordance rates for identical twins exceed 70%.

◇ Some racial groups have a very high incidence of type 2 diabetes; notable examples of this include the Pima Indians of Arizona (**42**) and South Sea Islanders, with prevalence rates of up to 50%.

◇ In the UK, the prevalence of type 2 diabetes among people of South Asian extraction is approximately three times that among those of European origin. Afro-Caribbeans show an intermediate prevalence (**43**). In the USA, Hispanic and Afro-Americans have higher rates of diabetes than those of European origin.

◇ The natural history of type 2 diabetes and its propensity to give rise to long-term complications also vary between races (examples being the relative lack of diabetic foot disease in British Asians and the high prevalence of diabetic nephropathy among those of Afro-Caribbean descent).

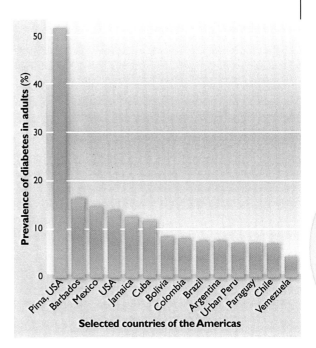

42 Genetic versus environmental factors. The Pima Indians of Arizona have the highest prevalence of type 2 diabetes in the world, far higher than other American populations. A homogeneous group, they have been extensively studied. There is an increased prevalence among Native Americans in general, possibly due to the interaction of genetic predisposition and a change from traditional diets. Genetically similar Pimas in Mexico, among whom the prevalence of obesity is less, are also much less susceptible to diabetes.

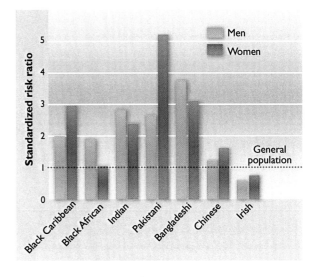

43 Ethnic minorites in England (2004). All minority ethnic groups, except Irish, have a higher standardized risk of (doctor-diagnosed) diabetes compared to the general population, with Pakistani women being particularly vulnerable.

Type 2 diabetes

Type 2 diabetes

- In most patients with type 2 diabetes, the pattern of inheritance suggests a polygenic disorder, with an important role for environmental factors (**44**) such as obesity and a low level of exercise. The specific genes already associated with the disease are, by and large, genes associated with reduced insulin secretion. A few genes, such as the fused-toe gene (FTO) have a modest effect leading to obesity, in the case of FTO probably due to increased food intake.
- Most recognized genes increase type 2 diabetes risk by 10–20% (OR 1.1–1.2), compared to obesity 510% (OR 5.1).
- Molecular biological techniques have not yet shown type 2 diabetes to be consistently associated with any abnormalities of the DNA coding for insulin, the insulin receptor or glucose transporter peptides (except in a small percentage [<5%] of cases). Abnormalities of the glucokinase gene and of certain hepatic nuclear factor genes cause some cases of MODY (see **10**), but not typical type 2 diabetes.

Associated conditions

- In Western populations, type 2 diabetes usually forms part of a syndrome of morphological and metabolic abnormalities. Some of these associations are referred to as 'metabolic syndrome' (see p. 50).
- The metabolic features of type 2 diabetes include fasting hyperinsulinemia, hyperglycemia, dyslipidemia, and high circulating concentrations of lactate, pyruvate, and glucogenic amino acids.
- Other associated conditions include hypertension, hyperuricemia, high plasma androgen:estrogen ratios, hypercoagulability of blood, endothelial dysfunction, and accelerated atherosclerosis.

44 The etiology of type 2 diabetes. Interaction between genes and the environment can lead to obesity/insulin resistance. Genetically susceptible β cells are unable to compensate for the increased secretory demand, resulting in dysfunction and cell death. *Adapted from Kahn, Hull, et al, 2006.*

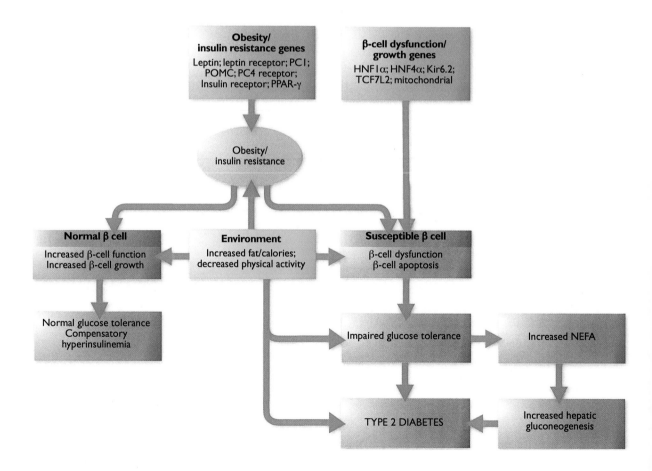

◇ A higher prevalence of and mortality from obesity- and alcohol-related cancers, such as pancreatic and liver cancers, have been observed in type 2 diabetes. However, this observation may be due to confounding factors and not diabetes *per se*.

Hyperinsulinemia and hyperglycemia

◆ The typical natural history of type 2 diabetes is reflected in a progressive decline in insulin secretory capacity, so that the metabolic picture changes over a period of years (**45**).

  ◇ Patients become insulin resistant, almost always because of obesity and physical inactivity.

  ◇ Insulin resistance causes the patient to progress over the years through a phase of hyperinsulinemia ('metabolic syndrome', 'insulin resistance syndrome').

  ◇ The hyperinsulinemia puts a strain on the β cells and progressive pancreatic failure is added to the pathophysiology.

  ◇ Thereafter, the patient proceeds through phases of increasingly severe hyperglycemia. At first, the glycemic defect will be subtle, such as IGT or IFG, but will then become Type 2 diabetes.

◆ Initially, therapy for type 2 diabetes may involve just lifestyle interventions, but, typically, oral hypoglycemic agents and, later, exogenous insulin will be needed as worsening β-cell failure supervenes.

Hypertension

◆ The association between diabetes and hypertension is strong and long recognized. The incidence of hypertension in obese patients with type 2 diabetes is about 50% in some series.

◆ Hypertension is associated with obesity and short stature in nondiabetic as well as diabetic groups.

◆ Diabetic patients are liable to develop the same secondary forms of hypertension as the nondiabetic population (and renal artery stenosis is commoner in diabetes), but most diabetic hypertensive patients have a low renin hypertension unlike that of nondiabetic patients with essential hypertension.

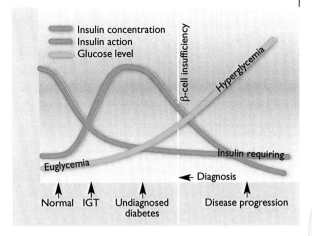

45 Natural history of type 2 diabetes. This model (the 'De Fronzo' hypothesis) shows that patients progress from normal glucose tolerance to IGT to diabetes. Though decreased insulin action is a contributor, it is the decline in β-cell production of insulin that heralds the onset of diabetes.

◆ In type 1 diabetes, hypertension is strongly linked with diabetic nephropathy. Although it is often uncertain whether this is initially cause or effect, it becomes a vicious cycle.

  ◇ There appear to be familial effects, with non-diabetic relatives of diabetic nephropathic hypertensive patients showing defects in ion transport function (erythrocyte Na^+/Li^+ counter transport and leukocyte Na^+/H^+ antiport) and an increased propensity to develop essential hypertension.

◆ Sodium retention and impaired natriuresis are characteristically found in both type 1 and type 2 hypertensive patients; exchangeable body sodium is increased by an average of 10%; this may be seen even before the development of any clinically detectable complications of diabetes.

  ◇ Possible mechanisms include increased glomerular filtration of glucose leading to enhanced proximal tubule sodium–glucose co-transport, hyperinsulinemia-induced over-activity of tubular sodium transporters, an extravascular shift of fluid with sodium and, in later stages, renal impairment.

Hypertension is common in type 2 diabetes patients and is often refractory to treatment.

Type 2 diabetes

- ◇ In glycemically-controlled type 1 and type 2 patients, plasma renin activity, angiotensin II, aldosterone and catecholamine concentrations are usually normal.
- ◇ Conversely, plasma atrial natriuretic peptide concentrations tend to be increased, and an exaggerated vascular reactivity to norepinephrine and angiotensin II is common, even in uncomplicated types 1 and 2 diabetes.

- Data from the UKPDS confirm that hypertension in type 2 diabetes is often refractory to treatment and a combination of anti-hypertensive agents is typically required to maintain 'good' blood pressure (BP) control. This study also made clear the relationship between BP and diabetic nephropathy, showing that a modest reduction in BP reduced the incidence of nephropathy and death.

Abnormalities of lipid metabolism

- Diabetes is associated with abnormalities of lipid metabolism. Several mechanisms have been suggested for these associations.
  - ◇ The obesity and body fat distribution common in type 2 diabetes are linked with dyslipidemias in nondiabetic subjects.
  - ◇ Nonenzymatic glycation of apolipoproteins impairs lipoprotein clearance.
  - ◇ Insulin is the principal regulator of lipolysis and, without its action, NEFA release from adipose tissue may be increased.
  - ◇ Much of this extra NEFA will be re-esterified by the liver to VLDL-triglyceride (see p.55).
  - ◇ Peripheral VLDL-triglyceride clearance may be impaired because insulin is needed to synthesize and secrete lipoprotein lipase, the principal enzyme responsible for clearing VLDL-triglyceride in some tissues.
  - ◇ Insulin also promotes LDL receptor function.
- Poor glycemic control in type 1 diabetes is associated with high concentrations of VLDL-cholesterol, LDL-cholesterol and total triglycerides, and sometimes with low HDL-cholesterol. Adequate insulin therapy usually leads to a fall in total triglyceride, and abnormalities of VLDL and LDL also improve. Patients with well-controlled type 1 diabetes can achieve plasma lipid concentrations similar to those of nondiabetic subjects; HDL may even be elevated.

Abnormalities of lipid metabolism are frequently present in patients with diabetes.

- Type 2 diabetes is strongly associated with low HDL-cholesterol, yet high VLDL-cholesterol and elevated triglyceride concentrations. Total cholesterol is often normal, but HDL:LDL or HDL:total cholesterol ratios are low.
  - ◇ In type 2 diabetes, the composition of VLDL particles changes, with more triglyceride and cholesterol ester relative to the apoprotein content.
  - ◇ LDL particles are typically small and dense.
  - ◇ These abnormalities are particularly atherogenic and there is a need to consider the HDL and triglycerides, rather than just total or LDL cholesterol, in the treatment of dyslipidemia in type 2 diabetes.
  - ◇ Improved glycemic control only partially improves the dyslipidemia of type 2 diabetes.

The metabolic syndrome and obesity

- Many of the associated features of type 2 diabetes co-segregate in members of a population even in nondiabetic subjects. Various overlapping syndromes have been introduced to reflect this fact, e.g. 'syndrome X', 'insulin resistance syndrome', 'metabolic syndrome'.
- Subjects with glucose intolerance (type 2 diabetes or IGT), fasting hyperinsulinemia, hypertriglyceridemia (mainly VLDL-triglyceride), low HDL cholesterol and hypertension have an increased predisposition to atherosclerosis and were said to have 'syndrome X'.
- 'Metabolic syndrome' is the more frequently discussed syndrome and includes abdominal obesity, but no formal requirement for insulin resistance. There has been debate on the cut-off points for the presence or absence of these features, and on the number of features required before an individual is labeled as having these related syndromes (**46**).

Definitions of metabolic syndrome

	IDF (2006)	WHO (1999)	EGIR (1999)	AHA/NCEP (2004)
Qualifying criteria	Central obesity (defined as waist circumference with ethnicity-specific values) AND any two of the other factors below	Presence of either: diabetes ; impaired glucose tolerance; impaired fasting glucose; OR insulin resistance AND any two of the other factors below.	Insulin resistance (defined as the top 25% of the fasting insulin values among nondiabetic individuals) AND any two of the other factors below	Any three of the factors below
Central obesity	As above. NB: If BMI is >30 kg/m², central obesity can be assumed and waist circumference does not need to be measured	Waist:hip ratio of males: >0.90; females: >0.85 AND/OR BMI >30 kg/m²	Waist circumference of males: ≥94 cm; females: ≥80 cm	Waist circumference of males: ≥102 cm; females: ≥88 cm
Triglycerides	Levels of >1.7 mmol/l (150.5 mg/dl) OR specific treatment for this lipid abnormality	Dyslipidemia counts as one criterion: triglyceride levels of ≥1.695 mmol/l (150 mg/dl)	Dyslipidemia counts as one criterion: triglyceride levels of ≥2.0 mmol/l (177 mg/dl)	Levels of ≥1.7 mmol/l (150.5 mg/dl)
High-density lipoprotein cholesterol (HDL)	Levels of <1.03 mmol/l (39.8 mg/dl) (males); <1.29 mmol/l (49.8 mg/dl) (females) OR specific treatment for this lipid abnormality	AND HDL levels of 0.9 mmol/l (34.7 mg/dl) (males); 1.0 mmol/l (38.6 mg/dl) (females)	AND/OR HDL levels of <1.0 mmol/l (38.6 mg/dl) OR treated for dyslipidemia	Levels of males: <1.03 mmol/l; females: <1.29 mmol/l
Blood pressure (BP)	Systolic BP of >130 mmHg OR diastolic BP of >85 mmHg OR treatment of previously diagnosed hypertension	Levels of ≥140/90 mmHg	Levels of ≥140/90 mmHg OR treatment of previously diagnosed hypertension	Levels of ≥130/85 mmHg OR treatment of previously diagnosed hypertension
Fasting plasma glucose (FPG)	Levels of >5.6 mmol/l (100 mg/dl) OR previously diagnosed type 2 diabetes	As above	Levels of ≥6.1 mmol/l (110 mg/dl)	Levels of ≥5.6 mmol/l (100 mg/dl) OR use of medication for hyperglycemia
Microalbuminuria		Urinary albumin excretion ratio of ≥20 mg/min OR albumin:creatinine ratio of ≥30 mg/g		

◇ Not all components are measured in routine clinical practice and the labels have no especial management implications. Some workers specifically exclude obese subjects from syndrome X but there are many features in common between slim subjects with syndrome X and those who are obese with metabolic syndrome.

46 **Metabolic syndrome.** People with metabolic syndrome have a five-fold greater risk of developing type 2 diabetes. The International Diabetes Federation (IDF) and the National Cholesterol Education Program (NCEP) have both recently issued updated diagnosis guidelines.

Type 2 diabetes

Insulin resistance is a prominent feature of obesity, especially of the android type. Obesity provokes compensatory hyperinsulinemia and the dyslipidemia and hypertension associated with obesity may follow from the insulin abnormalities. Obesity is a powerful indicator of type 2 diabetes risk (**47**).

Development of type 2 diabetes

Glucoregulatory defects in type 2 diabetes

◆ The causes of type 2 diabetes are partially understood.
  ◇ Reduced insulin secretion plays a major role, together with reduced insulin sensitivity.
  ◇ Hyperglycemia is due to elevated hepatic glucose output and (to a lesser extent) failure of skeletal muscle to take up glucose and store it as glycogen.
  ◇ There are also abnormalities in metabolic fluxes (**48**).

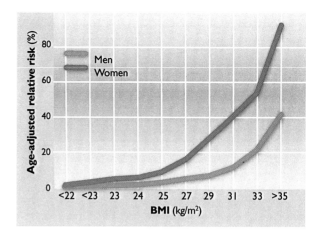

47 Obesity and diabetes. The link between obesity and type 2 diabetes is firmly established.

Pancreatic β-cell deficiency

◆ The importance of β-cell deficiency varies in different groups and individual cases of type 2 diabetes. In general, the β-cell deficiency becomes more severe with time (see p. 48). There are abnormalities of insulin secretion in all these patients, but the causes of these defects are not yet established.
  ◇ In individual patients it is often difficult to define the severity of the insulin secretory defect. Although β-cell dysfunction may be the prime abnormality in some cases of type 2 diabetes, usually the β-cell dysfunction is more subtle than in type 1 diabetes and is secondary to the preceding insulin resistance.
◆ The finding of marked insulin deficiency in an apparent type 2 patient should provoke a consideration of whether they are actually a LADA patient.
  ◇ Fortunately, the accurate distinction between insulin-deficient type 2 diabetes and late-onset type 1 diabetes often has few implications for the clinical management of individual patients.

Metabolic fluxes in insulin resistance syndrome/early type 2 diabetes

	CONCENTRATION	FLUX
Glucose	Increased fasting concentration	Normal whole body disposal rate; normal whole body glucose production and clearance
NEFA	Variable	Usually normal fasting total body production; impaired responsiveness to meal
VLDL	Increased concentration	Increased production, increased plasma half-life and increased whole body clearance
Oxidized fuel	Whole body respiratory quotient* reflects diet	Whole body respiratory quotient reflects diet, but seems to be higher in diabetes

*Respiratory quotient is the ratio of oxygen consumption to carbon dioxide production during biological oxidation at tissue level.

48 Alterations in metabolic fluxes. Insulin resistance causes increased flux of free fatty acids, leading to increased VLDL synthesis in the liver.

◆ Some patients with type 2 diabetes, especially obese subjects with mild glucose intolerance, may have hyperinsulinemia throughout the whole 24 hours.

◇ Some patients can exhibit both insulinopenia and hyperinsulinemia (relative to normal weight controls) at different times during a single day.

◇ It is fairly common to have fasting hyperinsulinemia combined with reduced β-cell reserve, relative to healthy subjects.

◆ The time course of insulin secretion in type 2 diabetes is abnormal, with patients typically exhibiting relative insulin deficiency during both the early phase of insulin secretion after an oral glucose load or meal and the first-phase insulin response to an intravenous glucose load. This loss of early insulin response to glucose is paralleled by defects in the pulsatility of insulin secretion.

◆ Insulin clearance is thought to be normal in type 2 diabetes, so hyperinsulinemia is a reflection of true hypersecretion. This hypersecretion represents a load on the pancreas and explains why increased concentrations of insulin precursors (such as pro-insulins) are seen in type 2 patients.

◆ However, over time, even patients who were hyperinsulinemic at diagnosis become progressively more insulin deficient. Such patients, together with those who are insulin deficient from diagnosis, often need exogenous insulin treatment to maintain near-normal glycemia. These patients may then be termed 'insulin-treated' or 'insulin-requiring', but it should be recognized that such insulin-*treated* patients form a heterogeneous group, very different in character from type 1, insulin-*dependent* patients.

Insulin resistance

◆ In 1970, Berson and Yalow defined insulin resistance as 'a state in which greater than normal amounts of insulin are required to elicit a quantitatively normal response.'

◆ Following the discovery of insulin in 1922, it was widely assumed that diabetes was due exclusively to a deficiency in insulin secretion. The concept of insulin resistance arose in the 1930s when Himsworth noted that the same amount of exogenous insulin injected into different diabetic subjects had different anti-hyperglycemic effects. Those with lesser anti-hyperglycemic responses were termed insulin-insensitive (or insulin-resistant). When the development of radio-immunoassay showed that many patients with type 2 diabetes had high levels of circulating insulin, the concept of insulin resistance was reinforced. Such patients are hyperglycemic, and hence by definition relatively insulin-deficient, yet they actually have more immunoreactive insulin than other people, such that their true 'insulin requirement' was believed to be larger still.

◆ Hyperinsulinemia with eu- or hyperglycemia is taken to indicate insulin resistance, since hyperinsulinemia produces hypoglycemia in subjects with normal insulin sensitivity.

◆ As insulin has several actions, resistance to insulin action may take several forms:

◇ Some subjects show resistance to hepatic effects.

◇ Some show resistance to skeletal muscle effects. (Activation of muscle glycogen synthase by insulin is often defective.)

◇ Some show resistance to liporegulatory effects.

◇ The degree of resistance may be different for different actions of insulin so that some subjects may have marked liver insulin resistance but relatively normal lipids (or other combinations).

All patients with type 2 diabetes have some beta-cell deficiency, which often gets more severe with time.

Insulin resistance means that more insulin than normal is needed to exert the glucoregulatory effects.

- There is incomplete consensus as to the cellular mechanisms underlying insulin resistance in most patients with type 2 diabetes, though multiple mechanisms have been suggested:
  - ◇ Competition between carbohydrate and lipid fuels (Randle cycle hypothesis). High circulating concentrations of alternative fuels, such as triglycerides, NEFA, lactate and ketone bodies, compete with glucose for metabolism and, in their presence, glucose clearance will be reduced.
  - ◇ Some insulin resistance can be interpreted as a result of 'cellular satiety', seen whenever intracellular sensors, such as UDP glucosamine, detect overabundant energy supply.
  - ◇ Some insulin resistance is attributable to specific cellular abnormalities, such as reduced numbers of insulin receptors, reduced receptor function, dysfunction of second messenger systems, and intracellular antagonists of insulin effects.
- These different hypotheses are not necessarily mutually exclusive. Lipid fuel competition may contribute to cellular satiety and provoke specific second messenger changes.
- Most glucose clearance occurs independently of insulin. This insulin-independent glucose clearance is defective in type 2 diabetes and contributes to hyperglycemia. Reduced tissue blood flow, particularly within skeletal muscle, may also reduce clearance of plasma glucose in diabetes.

The role of amylin
- Amylin (also known as islet amyloid polypeptide, IAPP) is a 37-amino-acid peptide co-secreted with insulin by β cells in all subjects with intact insulin secretion (and so not those with type 1 diabetes or those type 2 patients with severe insulin deficiency). The amino acid structure has some homology with calcitonin gene-related peptide.
- Plasma concentrations of amylin are very low ($<10^{-10}$ molar) in both diabetic and non-diabetic subjects.
- There is no established physiological role for amylin in the systemic circulation, but it has been suggested that it may have a physiological role in the regulation of insulin secretion within the islet, or have some effects on bone metabolism.

- Pathophysiological roles of amylin include the suggestion that it may induce insulin resistance in skeletal muscle, but this only occurs at pharmacological concentrations.
- Amylin fibrils (with typical amyloid features of secondary protein structure and insolubility) are deposited in islet cells in conditions of excess insulin secretion (such as insulinoma) and in situations where insulin secretion may have initially been increased but has subsequently declined (such as old age and type 2 diabetes). The possible role of amylin in the islet damage of type 2 diabetes is under intensive investigation.

Glucotoxicity and lipotoxicity

Glucotoxicity
- It has long been known that acute elevation of plasma glucose concentrations is able to induce a state of insulin resistance, coupled with impairment of insulin secretion in response to glucose (**49**).
- In the presence of normal β-cell mass, transient elevation of plasma glucose to levels just above the physiological range potentiates insulin secretion in both humans and animals, but chronic hyperglycemia reduces insulin secretion.
- Conversely, strict metabolic control is able to induce improvements in both insulin secretion and sensitivity, although not usually to normality. It is likely that multiple mechanisms contribute to this effect, including:
  - ◇ Changes in the K_m of glucose sensing systems, such as glucokinase/hexokinase, which may lead to alteration of the dose–response curve of the islet cell to blood glucose concentrations.
  - ◇ Changes in the ratio of proinsulin to insulin secretion.
  - ◇ Alteration in the functional activity of the membrane sulfonylurea-sensitive K^+ channel.
- It is likely that the 'honeymoon period' often observed in new-onset type 1 diabetes is at least partly attributable to a reduction in glucotoxicity.

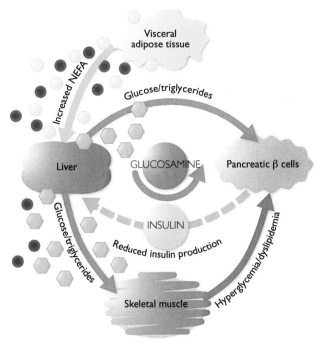

49 Glucotoxicity and lipotoxicity. Insulin resistance is related to elevated levels in the blood of both glucose and free fatty acids (NEFA). The metabolism of glucose to glucosamine is a possible unifying mechanism for both glucotoxicity and lipotoxicity, whereby the glucosamine pathway inhibits a number of steps in the insulin-signaling cascade.

◆ NEFA can induce insulin resistance in muscle via at least 3 putative mechanisms:
 ◇ The Randle cycle, mentioned above.
 ◇ Increased activity of protein kinase C via intermediates of fatty acid metabolism, such as diacyl glycerol, which promotes inactivating phosphorylation of the insulin receptor.
 ◇ NFκB activation, which has supposed vascular effects that might contribute to the observed increase in vascular damage preceding hyperglycemia.
◆ In the liver, NEFAs inhibit the suppression of glycogenolysis by insulin.
◆ Other mechanisms of lipotoxicity include modulation of adipocytokines, such as adiponectin, that could promote insulin resistance.
◆ Not all individuals with obesity and elevated NEFA rapidly develop diabetes. One explanation for this may lie in the fact that NEFAs are potent stimulators of insulin in normal individuals, an effect that might mitigate the tendency for NEFAs to induce insulin resistance. However, in subjects with type 2 diabetes and in their normoglycemic first-degree relatives, NEFAs do not induce a sufficient compensatory rise in insulin secretion to overcome the induced insulin resistance. Thus NEFAs may be able to cause diabetes in those with a genetic predisposition to β-cell dysfunction, but not in those with full β-cell reserve.
◆ PPARγ activators (see p. 146) may alleviate several of these NEFA-induced abnormalities by reducing plasma NEFA levels, increasing adiponectin and redistributing fat from visceral to subcutaneous deposits, thus reducing the direct effects on the liver and elsewhere.

Lipotoxicity
◆ Although adipose tissue has a large number of functions related to thermoinsulation, immunity, fertility, and protection of structures such as the eye, its main function is the uptake of energy during the postprandial state, energy storage in the form of tryglyderides, and the release of lipids in the form of NEFA in the fasting state (**49**).
◆ The consequences of an accumulation of lipids in nonadipose tissues include hepatic steatosis, lipid-induced cardiomyopathy, insulin resistance, and type 2 diabetes. This process is termed lipotoxicity.
◆ In fatless rodents and humans with generalized lipodystrophy there can be an especially severe form of lipotoxicity (including lipoapoptosis where programmed cell death occurs). This severe form is reversible in rodents by the transplantation of small amounts of normal adipose tissue into fatless rodents, but not by the transplantation of adipose tissue from *ob/ob* mice, which lack the ability to secrete leptin.
 ◇ In humans with generalized lipodystrophy, long-term treatment with leptin improves insulin resistance, hyperlipidemia and hepatic steatosis dramatically.

Very high plasma glucose concentrations can induce a state of insulin resistance.

Screening and prevention

◆ IGT, as defined by the National Diabetes Data Group and the WHO, is recognized as a high-risk state for type 2 diabetes. The standard definition has been updated on several occasions, but the evidence remains that IGT is a powerful predictor of diabetes progression, with a concomitant increased risk for macrovascular disease.

◆ IGT is common, affecting up to 25% of adults in the UK and USA.

◆ Several additional factors determine the risk of progression from IGT to type 2 diabetes: family history of diabetes, age, central and total obesity, physical inactivity, fetal maturation, and ethnic origin. The risk of progression to diabetes is greater for those with IGT than for those with IFG (**50**).

◆ As with type 2 diabetes, IGT is an insulin-resistant state and subjects have a reduced early-phase insulin response to intravenous or oral glucose challenge. It follows that glucose tolerance, as with diabetes, can be improved by improving insulin sensitivity and insulin secretion.

◇ Following intervention to reduce weight, reduce calorie intake, and increase exercise, middle-aged subjects with IGT have been successfully treated with these lifestyle changes with or without metformin, acarbose, orlistat, troglitazone, simvastatin, and angiotensin-converting enzyme inhibitors. For example, lifestyle changes (diet and exercise) reduced the 4-year incidence of diabetes by 58% in middle-aged, obese, IGT subjects in one study; by 58% in similar subjects by 3 years in another study; and by 31% by 3 years with metformin.

◇ The prospect of population screening for IGT is daunting, but the potential for successful therapeutic intervention is there.

50 **Prevention of type 2 diabetes.** Screening and Identification of those most at risk is the first step in preventing type 2 diabetes. There is convincing evidence that lifestyle modification is the most effective tool in preventing or delaying its onset, with moderate weight loss and physical activity substantially reducing the risk. However, some patients will also require pharmacologic intervention.

IGT is a powerful predictor of diabetes progression.

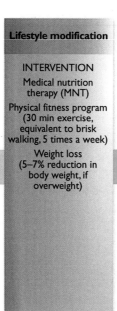

Early identification of risk

RISK FACTORS (AGE ≥30 IF HIGH RISK)

Family history of diabetes

Overweight

Sedentary lifestyle

Higher-risk ethnic origin

Previously identified IGT or IFG

Hypertension

Elevated triglycerides, low HDL, or both

History of gestational diabetes

Delivery of a baby of >4 kg (9 lb)

Severe psychiatric illness

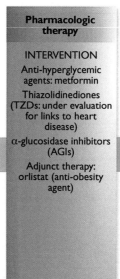

Lifestyle modification

INTERVENTION

Medical nutrition therapy (MNT)

Physical fitness program (30 min exercise, equivalent to brisk walking, 5 times a week)

Weight loss (5–7% reduction in body weight, if overweight)

Pharmacologic therapy

INTERVENTION

Anti-hyperglycemic agents: metformin

Thiazolidinediones (TZDs: under evaluation for links to heart disease)

α-glucosidase inhibitors (AGIs)

Adjunct therapy: orlistat (anti-obesity agent)

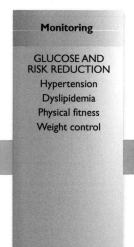

Monitoring

GLUCOSE AND RISK REDUCTION

Hypertension

Dyslipidemia

Physical fitness

Weight control

- Type 2 diabetes can be predicted using diabetes-associated conditions such as obesity, presence of IGT, and metabolic syndrome.
  - ◇ Evidence from long-term trials suggests that lifestyle interventions are more effective in the prevention of type 2 diabetes than the drugs tested. This may be expected since lifestyle intervention focuses on the pathogenetic mechanisms underlying the development of type 2 diabetes, in particular factors causing insulin resistance.
  - ◇ Theoretically, it would be possible to delay over 70% of cases of type 2 diabetes in persons at increased risk, if they were able to maintain normal body weight and engage in physical activity throughout their lives.
  - ◇ More than preventing diabetes, a healthy diet and lifestyle could prevent or retard heart disease.

Type 2 diabetes prevention studies

- Type 2 diabetes may be prevented or at least delayed by relatively modest degrees of weight loss and exercise. The interventions have involved individual counseling regarding weight loss, total fat intake, saturated fat intake, fiber intake, and physical exercise.
  - ◇ In recent studies, lifestyle interventions resulting in average weight loss of <7 kg over 6 months with some later regain resulted in a 58% reduction in cumulative diabetes incidence in the intervention groups during the period of the studies.
- There is evidence that tablet therapy can be beneficial in reducing progression to diabetes, especially in younger subjects; tablets that have been used successfully include metformin, rosiglitazone, acarbose, orlistat, and simvastatin.
- For patients unable to lose weight after appropriate lifestyle interventions, treatment with metformin may bring about a modest reduction in the incidence of type 2 diabetes.
- Other studies have shown that adopting a more physically active lifestyle appears to confer useful protection independently of body weight. Several trials have shown successful prevention or delay of progression from a state of IGT to type 2 diabetes by adopting different interventions (**51, 52**).

Trials determining prevention/delay of progression from IGT to type 2 diabetes

Lifestyle change trials	Risk reduction vs placebo (%)
Malmö study	63
Da Qing study	42
Finnish Diabetes Prevention Study (DPS)	58
Diabetes Prevention Program (DPP)	58

Medication trials	
TRIPOD: troglitazone	55
STOP-NIDDM: acarbose	25
XENDOS: orlistat	37
DPP: metformin	75
DREAM: rosiglitazone and ramipril	60
NAVIGATOR: nateglinide/valsartan	0/14

51 **Type 2 diabetes prevention studies.** Several long-term trials have studied the effectiveness of a range of medications as well as lifestyle changes: lifestyle change and glitazones have proved the most successful, although both troglitazone and rosiglitazone have since been withdrawn due to concerns over side-effects.

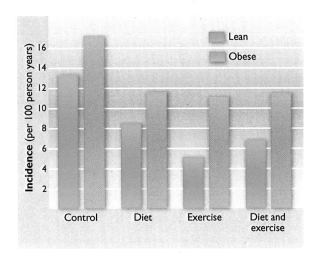

52 **Lifestyle interventions.** The Da Qing study examined the effect over 6 years of diet and exercise intervention in Chinese subjects with IGT and a mean age of 45. The diet intervention saw a 31% reduction in the risk of developing type 2 diabetes, while exercise or exercise combined with diet showed a 46% reduction and a 42% reduction, respectively.

Type 2 diabetes

CHAPTER 5

Diabetes screening and patient care

Management overview

- The goals of diabetes management are, at first glance, easily established. We know that the excess mortality associated with diabetes is due to macrovascular disease. The morbidity due to diabetes results from both macrovascular and microvascular disease. The aim of therapy is to normalize excess mortality and morbidity, so therapy should be aimed at risk factors for both macrovascular and microvascular diseases.
  - ◇ Modifiable risk factors for macrovascular disease are hypertension, hypercholesterolemia, obesity, smoking, and hyperglycemia.
  - ◇ Risk factors for microvascular disease are largely the same, but predominantly hyperglycemia and hypertension.
  - ◇ Since many type 2 diabetic patients have a combination of these risk factors, many patients will require a combination of drugs to manage their diabetes.
  - ◇ In type 1 diabetes, insulin therapy is mandatory once insulin dependence is established, and in these patients the focus is much more on management of glycemia, as these patients are generally younger and have fewer modifiable risk factors than patients with type 2 diabetes.
- The management of type 2 diabetes is complex and the physician will have to consider the interplay between the psychosocial background, various risk factors, and several therapeutic agents before deciding on a regimen appropriate to the patient. In practical terms the therapy of type 2 diabetes involves a trade-off between what is desirable and what is practically possible.

- Different studies of treatment, including the UKPDS and DCCT, illustrate the significant benefits that may be achieved by appropriate treatment. Cost/benefit assessments indicate that improved diabetes care compares favorably with other established healthcare programs, such as breast cancer screening.
- New drugs promise a substantial expansion of the current, rather limited, therapeutic options.
- An increasing appreciation of the importance of patient education suggests that these new medications can translate into real benefit for the patient.

Risk factors

- Patients with type 2 diabetes have an increased mortality (up to four times that of the nondiabetic population) attributed mainly to macrovascular disease, notably cardiovascular disease.
- Diabetes in developed countries is the commonest single cause of limb amputations, the commonest cause of blindness in working life, and the commonest cause of renal failure.
- The macrovascular disease risk is associated with smoking, lack of exercise, hypertension, obesity, dyslipidemia, and hyperglycemia. This network of risk factors, when it occurs concurrently, is called the metabolic or insulin-resistance syndrome, since all these factors are associated with insulin resistance and can precede type 2 diabetes (see also pp.50–52).
  - ◇ Metabolic syndrome may be present in up to 25% of the nondiabetic population and, in adult life, about 2–12% per year of these individuals progress to diabetes.

Annual examination

- Diabetes patients should be reviewed, at the very least once per year, by:
  - ◇ Their general practitioner.
  - ◇ A diabetes center (which is often attached to a hospital).
  - ◇ A hospital clinic.
  - ◇ OR a combination of these three.
- All diabetes patients should have access to advice outside the routine general practitioner clinic.
- The purposes of a diabetes clinic are to:
  - ◇ Optimize therapy (e.g. targets set for risk factors).
  - ◇ Provide patient education.
  - ◇ Screen for diabetes complications.
  - ◇ Treat established or developing complications.
- Monitoring of therapy includes assessment of:
  - ◇ Weight.
  - ◇ Height (using centile charts for children).
  - ◇ Urine (checking for ketones, albumin, and, in young adults and children, micro-albuminuria).
  - ◇ HbA1c, blood glucose, lipid profile, creatinine.
  - ◇ Blood pressure.
  - ◇ Smoking.
- There are key areas to be considered when examining a patient with diabetes (**53**).

Diabetes patients should be reviewed at least once per year.

Since prevention of complications is better and easier than cure, early referral is preferable.

---

53 Examination of a diabetic patient. It is specifically important to look out for potential causes of secondary diabetes and diabetes-associated microvascular and macro-vascular changes.

Screening for complications

Eyes

- Determine visual acuity. This can be done using the commonly used Snellen's chart.
- Extraocular eye movements can also be checked at this time.
- Dilate pupils 30 minutes before the eye is examined with a mydriatic, such as tropicamide 0.5%.
  - ◇ Dilating drugs should not be used in patients with a history of glaucoma, except with the advice of an ophthalmologist.
- *Ophthalmoscopy* is used to carry out a systematic examination of the eyes (**54**):
  - ◇ The ophthalmologic examination begins at an arm's length. At this distance, cataracts are silhouetted against the red reflex of the retina.

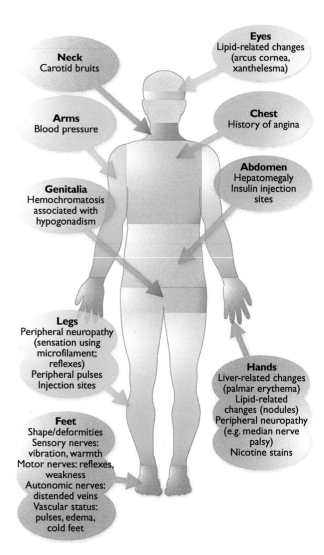

Neck
Carotid bruits

Arms
Blood pressure

Genitalia
Hemochromatosis associated with hypogonadism

Eyes
Lipid-related changes (arcus cornea, xanthelesma)

Chest
History of angina

Abdomen
Hepatomegaly
Insulin injection sites

Legs
Peripheral neuropathy (sensation using microfilament; reflexes)
Peripheral pulses
Injection sites

Feet
Shape/deformities
Sensory nerves: vibration, warmth
Motor nerves: reflexes, weakness
Autonomic nerves: distended veins
Vascular status: pulses, edema, cold feet

Hands
Liver-related changes (palmar erythema)
Lipid-related changes (nodules)
Peripheral neuropathy (e.g. median nerve palsy)
Nicotine stains

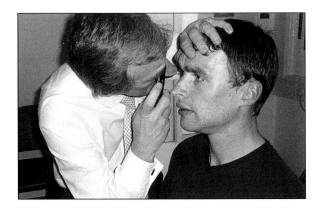

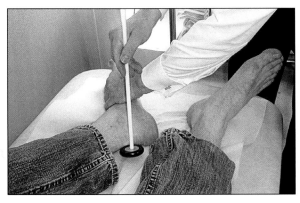

54, 55 Screening for complications. Indirect ophthalmoscopy and ankle-reflex testing.

◇ The ophthalmoscope is advanced until the retina is in focus. Examination of the retina begins at the optic disc, moves through each quadrant in turn, and ends with the macula (since this is least comfortable for the patient) by requesting the patient to look into the light.

◇ The ophthalmoscope is then adjusted to the +10 diopter lens for examination of the cornea, anterior chamber, and lens.

◇ Fundal photography, graded by a trained individual, is increasingly being used to screen fundi for retinopathy.

◆ Patients with retinopathy should be examined regularly by a diabetologist or an ophthalmologist. The following circumstances dictate immediate referral to an ophthalmologist:

◇ Deteriorating visual acuity.

◇ Hard exudates encroaching on the macula.

◇ Pre-proliferative changes (cotton-wool spots or venous beading).

◇ New vessel formation.

Kidneys

◆ Urine is tested for protein using a dipstick. Remember that trace positive is not positive if fresh urine is being used for the test.

◆ Some centers check for microalbuminuria, which can also be done using a dipstick.

◇ This is valid as a marker of early kidney disease in children and young adults only when present on at least two separate occasions in an early morning urine sample.

◇ If microalbuminuria is confirmed, treatment with an angiotensin-receptor blocker (ARB) or angiotensin-converting enzyme (ACE) inhibitor should be started.

◆ Serum creatinine should be analyzed annually.

◆ Referral to a renal specialist is advised once the creatinine level has reached 150 µmol/l (1.7 mg/dl). An investigation and management plan should have been devised with the local clinic.

Feet

◆ Inspection of the feet is performed to identify anatomical distortions, pressure points, ulcers, injuries, or problems with footwear.

◆ Examination is carried out for blood supply (by checking peripheral pulses) and nerve supply (by checking peripheral sensation and reflexes [55]).

◆ Refer to a chiropodist if any problems are identified. Since prevention is better and easier than cure, early referral is preferable.

Erectile dysfunction

◆ History should assess whether the patient can get an erection, penetration or emission. Questions should be direct and unequivocal, as otherwise the response may not be informative.

◆ Examination should exclude hypogonadal features, small testes and penile changes, such as Peyronie's disease.

Vascular disease

◆ History should be assessed, e.g. pain in chest or legs, erectile dysfunction.

◆ Examination includes checking for bruit in carotids, palpating peripheral foot pulses.

◆ Special investigations may be necessary, e.g. an electrocardiogram (ECG).

◆ Refer to a cardiologist if there is either angina or cardiac dysfunction.

Diabetes screening and patient care

Treating children

Types of childhood diabetes

◆ Most children (under 18 years) have type 1 diabetes (**56**).

   ◇ As childhood obesity increases throughout the world an increasing proportion have type 2 diabetes (**57**).

   ◇ A small proportion will have maturity-onset diabetes of the young (MODY) (see pp.17 and 18).

   ◇ An even smaller proportion have neonatal diabetes, which may be permanent or transient, and predominates when diabetes is diagnosed before 2 years of age and especially within 6 months of birth.

56 **Childhood diabetes.** While type 1 diabetes accounts for most cases in children, in industrialized societies, type 2 is increasingly prevalent. MODY accounts for only 1% of cases.

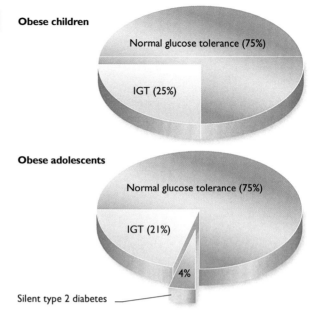

57 **Childhood obesity and IGT.** The prevalence of impaired glucose tolerance and type 2 diabetes in obese children and adolescents has been found to be high.

Diabetes in childhood

TYPE OF DIABETES	PRINCIPAL CAUSES
Type 1 diabetes	Autoimmune (see Chapter 3)
Type 2 diabetes	Decreased insulin secretion and obesity (see Chapter 4)
Maturity-onset diabetes of the young (MODY)	Dominantly inherited variant of type 2 diabetes mellitus (see Chapter 1)
Secondary diabetes Chromosomal abnormalities:	Down's syndrome Turner's syndrome Klinefelter's syndrome
Inherited disorders:	Prader–Willi syndrome Laurence–Moon–Biedl syndrome DIDMOAD syndrome Leprechaunism Lipodystrophy Ataxia–telangiectasia (Rabson) Mendenhall syndrome
Inherited disorder with pancreatic disease:	Cystic fibrosis Cystinosis Thalassemia
Acquired pancreatic disorders	Postpancreatectomy

◆ Type 1 diabetes is invariably treated with insulin.

◆ The optimal treatment of type 2 diabetes in children and adolescents remains to be determined. Common sense suggests that treatment regimens similar to those for adults with type 2 diabetes would be appropriate. However, many of these patients will be started on insulin initially on the assumption that they have type 1 diabetes, before the correct diagnosis is established.

◆ Treatment of MODY patients with oral agents often achieves excellent glycemic control, and the use of these agents in this context has been useful in confirming their long-term safety in younger patients. The physician should be alerted to MODY when there is a strong family history of diabetes.

◆ The causes of neonatal diabetes are predominantly genetic mutations in the sulfonylurea or potassium channels, so these children respond to sulfonylurea therapy.

Good glycemic control in the early years of diabetes may have a lasting effect on prevention of complications.

Management of young patients

◆ Management of children is not unlike management of the adult. However, it often requires particular sensitivity to the balance between the child's social independence and dependence on others. Younger children will be much more dependent on family and friends for supervision of their care. Developing independence as children get older is important for their ability to manage diabetes throughout their lifetime. Understanding and dealing in a sympathetic way with parents' understandable reluctance to cede too much independence is crucial to the management of teenage diabetes.

◆ Hypoglycemia is a particular problem in children, in whom the warning symptoms can differ from hypoglycemia in adults.

◆ Symptoms of note due to hypoglycemia in young children include:
  ◇ Bedwetting.
  ◇ Naughtiness.
  ◇ Tearfulness.
  ◇ Bad temper.
  ◇ Poor performance in school.

◆ Glycemic targets should be essentially the same as in adult patients (see pp. 132 and 133).

◆ Long-term follow-up of the young adults who constituted the DCCT cohort has suggested that good glycemic control in the early years of diabetes may have a lasting effect on prevention of complications, even when there is a subsequent modest decline in glycemic control. This study also showed for the first time that early glycemic control protects against cardiovascular disease later in life as well as microvascular disease. The DCCT did not specifically enroll patients who had developed diabetes in early childhood, but there is no reason to believe that the lessons from the study would not apply.
  ◇ It makes sense, therefore, to try to apply the same standards of care in childhood diabetes that we would strive for in more mature patients.

◆ Even when there is reason to question the level of competence for self-management among children with diabetes and their families, instruction on intensive insulin treatment can be very beneficial (**58**).

◆ Sometimes the fear of hypoglycemia limits attempts to obtain optimum diabetes control, and this is understandable.

◆ Optimal use of newer insulin analogs in 'basal and bolus' regimens, or of subcutaneous insulin infusion pumps (see p. 160), should enable most young diabetic people to achieve reasonably good control with less risk of hypoglycemia. Adolescents and many young children embrace the technologies of newer delivery devices and monitoring systems much more readily than older patients.

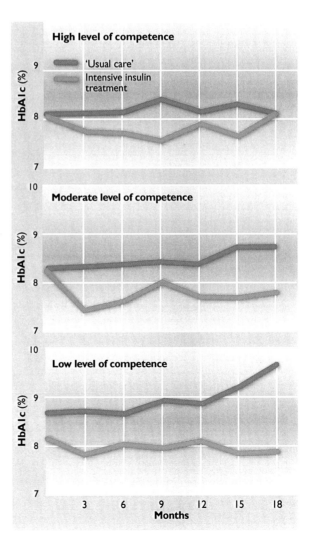

58 Diabetes self-management. In a study of 142 young people, intensive therapy gave improved glycemic control irrespective of self-management competence, but competence level was more significant with 'usual care'. *Adapted from Wysocki T et al, Diabetes Care, 2003.*

Diabetes screening and patient care

◇ In light of the potential long-term benefit of excellent glycemic control achieved *early* in the course of diabetes, every effort should be made to facilitate access to these newer technologies to as many children and adolescents with diabetes as possible.

◇ However, if optimum control is difficult, *any* reduction in HbA1c is associated with a marked decrease in complication risk. Thus, never abandon trying to get better control.

◆ Common issues regarding children with diabetes:

◇ Immunization programs in diabetic children are unaltered.

◇ Illness is no more prevalent in diabetic children, though urinary tract infection is more common.

◇ Bedwetting is no more prevalent in diabetic children but might be due to nocturnal hyperglycemia or hypoglycemia.

◇ Reluctance to take injections should be sympathetically handled and expert advice sought on needleless pens and injection technique.

◇ Hypoglycemia may present differently. Measure blood glucose if in doubt.

◇ Diet should be similar as for the rest of the family, and low in refined sugar. Try to keep meal times to a routine, but avoid being obsessive about this.

◇ Diabetic children should be encouraged to participate in all aspects of sport and play at school. Teachers may need to be advised.

◇ People around the child should be aware that the child has diabetes and what to do in case they develop hypoglycemic coma.

◇ Diabetes is an excellent opportunity for manipulative behavior. We all do it. But having diabetes is no excuse to live a different life.

◇ Linear growth is, on average, only slightly reduced in diabetes, especially in very young children with poor control. Puberty may also be delayed by 2 years or arrested. Both should be monitored (**59**) and if changes are noted then referral to a specialist may be required to exclude other causes (e.g. hypothyroidism, gluten enteropathy) and for therapy as required.

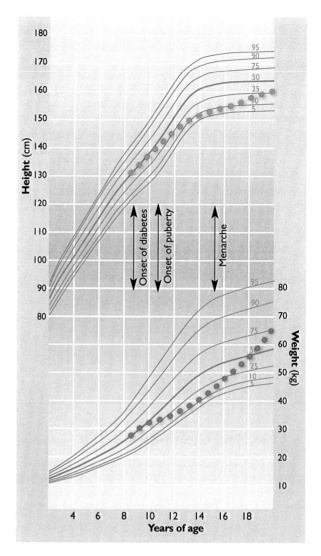

59 Growth and development. Height and weight increase with age in a child developing type 1 diabetes. This girl had poor glucose control post-diagnosis. Note the fall in both height and weight from the 60th centile to lower centiles after diagnosis, with a delay in both puberty and the onset of menarche. Note also the start of catch-up growth after menarche and the mismatch between weight and height associated with relative overweight thereafter.

Developing independence is important to enable children to manage diabetes throughout their lifetime.

The elderly diabetes patient

- The number of elderly people with diabetes has been increasing steadily.
  - ◇ Approximately 10% of people over 65 years of age have diagnosed diabetes and another 10% have undiagnosed hyperglycemia. In the US, total prevalence of DM (i.e. diagnosed plus undiagnosed) is 20.9% in those above 60 years.
  - ◇ It is estimated that by 2025 about a third of diabetic patients will be 75 years or older.
- In part, the increase in diabetes frequency is due to age-related changes in glucose metabolism, including decreased insulin secretion and decreased insulin sensitivity (**60**).
- Hyperglycemia in an elderly person is usually due to type 2 diabetes, but type 1 diabetes may also present late in life.
- Diabetes as a feature of underlying pancreatic cancer is more likely in the elderly, but accounts for only a small proportion of all cases of diabetes.
- Clinical presentation in older people may be 'atypical' and not as clear cut as in children or younger adults – for example, unexplained weight loss without other 'classic' symptoms of hyperglycemia.
- Hyperosmolar, nonketotic coma with extreme hyperglycemia, but no antecedent history of thirst or polyuria, may be a presenting feature of diabetes in the elderly, particularly in patients treated with diuretic drugs or steroids.
- As with children and adolescents, attention must be paid to achieving a balance between social autonomy and dependence. In principle, the aims of treatment are no different than in younger patients – relief of symptoms and prevention of complications.
- Macrovascular disease, hypertension, renal impairment, and failing vision due to macular degeneration or cataracts are all increasingly prevalent with advancing age regardless of diabetes, so efforts to combat the additional risk that diabetes presents in respect of these disabilities should be just as strenuous in the elderly as in younger people.

Management of elderly patients

- A number of factors in the elderly may interfere with compliance and complicate the management of patients:
  - ◇ Multiple pathologies and drug therapies can result in drug interactions and poor compliance. Compliance is related inversely to the number of drugs.
  - ◇ Drugs in the elderly are not metabolized so efficiently as in the young, and dosages may need to be lower.
- It may be considered necessary or prudent to identify the most important areas for intervention rather than identify all therapies required. There may be circumstances where intensifying treatment would not be expected to have a significant impact – or, worse, may have an adverse one – on a patient's overall sense of well-being or eventual outcome.

Diabetes screening and patient care

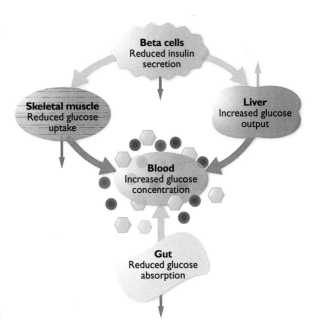

60 Glucose metabolism in the elderly. Decreased insulin secretion and sensitivity lead to raised glucose levels, despite reduced glucose absorption.

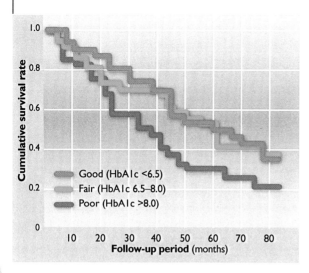

61 Glycemic control and survival rates. Survival rates in groups of diabetic patients on chronic hemodialysis over a 7-year period, indicating a better survival in patients with fair to good HbA1c levels. The average age of entry was over 60 years. *Adapted from Oomichi T et al, Diabetes Care, 2008.*

Control of hypoglycemia

◆ There is, however, the danger of acquiescing in the face of poor glycemic control or inadequate management of hypertension or hyperlipidemia in the mistaken belief that control of these risk factors for vascular disease is less worthwhile or effective in the elderly.

◇ A recent study from the Veterans Administration in the US confirmed that older patients and those with comorbid illnesses were least likely to have their therapy stepped up at outpatient clinic visits when glycemic control was clearly inadequate.

◇ In the absence of any study that proves the contrary, it is prudent to provide careful intensive outpatient management to elderly and more chronically ill patients as is offered to younger patients.

◇ It has been shown that poor glycemic control is an independent predictor of decreased survival in diabetic patients – many elderly – on hemodialysis (**61**), so it seems reasonable to assume a similar potential benefit in other situations of chronic ill health.

◇ A conscious decision to 'soft pedal' with regard to diabetes management in the elderly and infirm may contribute to their despondency or a sense of abandonment, at a time when they require exactly the opposite (**62, 63**).

◆ Strenuous efforts should be made to avoid hypoglycemia.

◇ Severe hypoglycemia is a hazard with longer-acting sulfonylureas such as chlorpropamide and glibenclamide in the elderly, especially when there is impairment of renal function; short-acting insulin secretagogues such as glipizide, gliclazide, repaglinide, or nateglinide are preferable.

◇ Noninsulinotropic agents, such as metformin, acarbose or thiazolidinediones (TZDs), are potentially safer in that on their own they are unlikely to cause hypoglycemia. However they are associated with other side-effects.

◇ Metformin should be used with caution in patients with impaired renal or cardiac function, because of the rare occurrence of lactic acidosis. Serum creatinine will often underestimate the degree of renal impairment in older, frail patients, and more use of formulae should be made, for example, estimated glomerular filtration rate (eGFR), the Cockcroft–Gault equation, or the Modification of Diet in Renal Disease (MDRD) formula.

◇ The glucose-dependent action of GLP-1 means that DPP-4 (dipeptidyl peptidase-4) inhibitors such as sitagliptin and saxagliptin have little inherent hypoglycemic risk; this makes these oral agents an attractive option in the elderly, though there are as yet relatively few long-term efficacy and safety data in the elderly population. Dose adjustment is required with impaired renal function.

◇ The GLP-1 agonists exenatide and liraglutide are also unlikely to cause hypoglycemia, but the initial frequency of gastrointestinal adverse effects is likely to make them less attractive in this population.

Management problems in the elderly

Living alone, poverty, poor diet – poor compliance

Intellectual impairment, depression, and dementia – poor compliance

Poor vision and dexterity – difficulty with blood test and injections

Coexisting diseases and drugs – potential for confusion and drug interaction

Multiple drug therapy – poor compliance

Decreased mobility and exercise – poor lifestyle

62 Management problems. Social, economic, and other health problems may lead to poor compliance with diabetes management among the elderly.

- Similar care to avoid hypoglycemia is required with insulin treatment in the elderly, but fear of hypoglycemia should not lead to avoidance of insulin treatment when it is clearly the most appropriate option.
  - ◇ Failing eyesight, decreased manual dexterity, and problems with memory may all be cited as barriers to insulin treatment; however, ways should be found to overcome such barriers when insulin treatment is essential or clearly better than other options.
  - ◇ Use of insulin glargine or detemir once a day may be sufficient to protect against ketoaci-dosis or hyperosmolar nonketotic coma if additional mealtime insulin is just not practical due to social circumstances.
  - ◇ When mealtime insulin is used, rapid-acting insulin analogs are preferred; timing of the injection is vitally important, either immedi-ately before or after the meal, with dosage adjustment if there is concern about ability to complete the meal, in order to avoid hypo-glycemia.
  - ◇ For similar reasons, it is probably better to avoid fixed-ratio mixed insulin, even though it may seem superficially attractive.
- It is worth considering that, for the person with limited social independence who nevertheless lives alone, the employment of a carer to give insulin will help prevent social isolation.

Therapy for diabetes in the elderly

Determine current quality of life and prognosis

Assess priorities in treating diabetes and other diseases

Avoid hypoglycemia

Treat diabetes according to individual targets

Screen for complications and treat to maintain quality of life

Be cautious with drug dosages and insulin use

63 Therapy key points. Therapy should be chosen based on the individual needs, wishes, and abilities of each patient.

Ethnic minorities

- Patients with diabetes should be treated in the same manner, irrespective of their race, and according to the type of diabetes and risk factors.
- The following points are of particular note:
  - ◇ There is wide variation in diabetes incidence according to race, both for type 1 and type 2.
  - ◇ Macrovascular disease is particularly prevalent in some ethnic groups such as Asian Indians.
  - ◇ Hyperosmolar nonketotic coma is more common in African-Americans than in people of European origin.
  - ◇ Hypertension in patients of African origin is often low-renin, which may explain why response to angiotensin-converting enzyme inhibitors is poor. Nevertheless, these agents, beta-adrenoreceptor blockers, and calcium channel blockers are the first choice (though evidence for the success of this strategy is lacking).
- The month of Ramadan poses a problem for prac-ticing Muslims on tablets or insulin. It is possible to obtain permission to break the fast for medical reasons, and patients should consult their holy leader if unsure. Alternatively, during daylight hours patients could avoid short-acting insulin and insulinotropic agents. The availability of the newer insulins, glargine and detemir, with little or

Diabetes screening and patient care

no peak action, should help to reduce the risks of hypoglycemia and dehydration. Hypoglycemia, if it does occur, is a justifiable reason to break the fast.

◇ During Ramadan, the diet changes as one only eats twice per day: at Sehri (before sunrise) and at Iftar (after sunset), but not between those times. Patients with diabetes should take Sehri just before sunrise and not earlier, and be very strict about avoiding sweet food.

◆ Patients of differing ethnicities have diverse dietary preferences, and one of the features of the ethnic heterogeneity of modern western society is the much greater variety of cuisine available to, and enjoyed by, all. It is important, therefore, that the nutritional advice offered takes into account the fact that many patients will not be following a traditional western-type diet.

The amount of time spent with an educator correlates with outcomes.

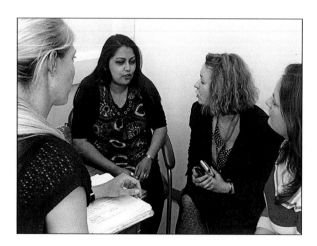

64 Patient care. Management involves a team: physician, dietitian, nurse specialist, and patient discuss a problem.

Patient education and community care

◆ The care of diabetes is based on self-management by the patient, who is advised by those with specialized knowledge.

◆ Education should begin when the patient is diagnosed.

◆ The diabetes team members include the patient, doctors, nurses, diabetes educators, dietitians, and chiropodists (**64**). Lack of motivation, expertise or education of any one of these individuals can disrupt the quality of care.

◆ A particular challenge is the diverse socio-economic and ethnic background of diabetic patients presenting to the educators. Culture-appropriate educational materials and illustrations, such as examples of carbohydrate servings and food groups, can be made more understandable and effective when adapted to the patient's local setting.

◆ Diabetes self-management education (DSME) is helpful, at least in the short term, in improving glycemic control and psychosocial outcomes in diabetic patients. The amount of time spent with the educator correlates with outcome.

◆ In the US, it is recommended that DSME programs fulfil the following:

◇ Describe the diabetes disease process and treatment options.
◇ Incorporate appropriate nutritional management into lifestyle.
◇ Incorporate physical activity into lifestyle.
◇ Use medications safely for maximum therapeutic effectiveness.
◇ Monitor blood glucose and other parameters and use the results for self-management decision-making.
◇ Prevent, detect, and treat acute complications.
◇ Prevent, detect, and treat chronic complications.
◇ Develop personal strategies to address psychosocial issues and concerns.
◇ Develop personal strategies to promote health and behavior change.

Living with diabetes

◆ There may be aspects of the lives of diabetes patients that have an influence on the choice of treatment (**65**).

Employment
◆ All jobs are open to people with diabetes except a few in which the risk of hypoglycemia, due to insulin therapy, might put others at risk (**66**).

Finance
◆ It is important that life and car insurance companies are informed of the diagnosis of diabetes or the start of insulin therapy.
  ◇ Some brokers and companies are more accommodating than others towards insuring patients with diabetes, and will offer better deals, though the premium will be dependent on the type of insurance, the nature of the therapy, the risk of hypoglycemia, and the presence of complications. Visual acuity and fields must be assessed to determine suitability for driving.
◆ In the UK, patients with diabetes are exempt from prescription charges; their general practitioner should sign an SP92 form to claim exemption.

Sport
◆ Having diabetes should rarely be a bar to participation in sport. People with diabetes can play, and many excel at, most sports.
◆ Some sports are wary of allowing patients on insulin to participate in competition such as scuba diving, motor rally driving, and boxing.
◆ Patients exercising intensively are at risk of hypoglycemia and should:
  ◇ Measure blood glucose before exercise (perhaps with a general rule of not starting exercise if blood sugar is less than 5.6 mmol/l [100 mg/dl] or greater than 14 mmol/l [250 mg/dl]).

66 Employment restrictions. Some occupations are exempt from disability discrimination legislation, usually where the risk of hypoglycemia would be dangerous.

Lifestyle problems

AREA	EXAMPLES
Employment	Shift-workers Long working day (resulting in early breakfast, late evening meal, or erratic meal times) Skipping midday meal or frequent business lunches International travel
Eating	National and cultural variations (e.g. time of main meal, varying dietary compositions) Individual variations (e.g. availability, preferences, affordability, dining out)
Exercise	Sportsmen and women Sedentary office workers Manual laborers
Travel	Long-haul air travel Means of traveling to work (e.g. cycling, long walks)
Leisure	Strenuous hobbies (e.g. sports, gardening)

65 Living with diabetes. The choice of treatment may need to take into account a patient's lifestyle.

Employment exclusions, UK and USA

EMPLOYMENT	EXAMPLES
Vocational driving	Large goods vehicle (LGV), passenger-carrying vehicles (PCV), locomotives or underground trains, professional drivers (chauffeurs), taxi drivers (variable, depending on local authority)
Civil aviation	Commercial pilots, flight engineers, aircrew, air-traffic controllers
National and emergency services	Armed forces (army, navy, air force), police force, fire brigade or rescue services, merchant navy, prison and security services
Dangerous work areas	Offshore oil-rig work, moving machinery, incinerator loading, hot-metal areas, railway tracks
Work at heights	Overhead linesmen, crane driving, scaffolding/high ladders or platforms

Diabetes screening and patient care

◇ Take 20 g carbohydrate every 45 minutes during exercise.

◇ Keep fast-acting glucose preparations (such as Dextrosol in Europe) in their pocket in case they feel hypoglycemic.

◇ Avoid dangerous situations, such as swimming alone.

Holidays and travel

◆ Patients with insulin-treated diabetes who are traveling will need:

◇ Insulin and insulin syringes, or pen devices or insulin pump supplies, and glucose-monitoring equipment. Bring spare insulin and syringes when possible in case one is mislaid. Insulin in various forms is widely available in most international destinations nowadays. Nevertheless it still makes sense to bring extra supplies for emergency, and people using pumps and pens should consider bringing spare 'traditional' vials of rapid-acting and basal insulin, and syringes.

◇ Identification to confirm that they have diabetes (e.g. Medic Alert bracelet) and letter to confirm they need to carry syringes/devices in aeroplanes. The US Transportation Security Administration allows the following through the checkpoint after screening: insulin if clearly identified, syringes when accompanied by insulin or other injectables, insulin pumps, and other supplies (**67**).

◇ Glucose tablets to manage or avoid hypoglycemia.

◇ Medical insurance.

◆ Vaccinations should be done as required, there are no special needs when someone has diabetes.

◆ On the day of travel aim particularly to avoid hypoglycemia, as this can be very disruptive to travel arrangements; so plan to check glucose levels frequently:

◇ When traveling eastwards, the day is shorter, so the insulin dose may need to be reduced, and extra snacks may be required. Plan to resume the usual insulin schedule, fitting in with the times in the particular time zone, once at the destination.

◇ When traveling westwards, the day is longer and an additional insulin injection may be required; use soluble (regular insulin in the US) or rapid-acting insulin for the extra injection, take an additional meal, and monitor the blood glucose carefully. Again, resume the usual schedule in the new time zone.

◇ If the trip is very long, perhaps with stopovers, a change in regime may be necessary so that it is possible to use soluble (regular) or rapid-acting insulin before each meal.

Driving

◆ Patients with diabetes who drive a car or want to drive a car must:

◇ Inform their car insurers as soon as they have been diagnosed; not to do so could invalidate any insurance. Check with other insurance brokers if the insurance premiums are increased following the diagnosis of diabetes; be prepared to 'shop around'.

◇ Inform the licensing authority (in the UK the DVLA; in the US, relevant state agency) if you are treated with tablets or insulin.

◇ The DVLA will ask the patient to sign a declaration allowing their doctor to disclose medical information about them if they are treated with insulin. This point applies to motorcyclists and car drivers. Licenses restricted to 1, 2 or 3 years only are provided if diabetes is treated with insulin.

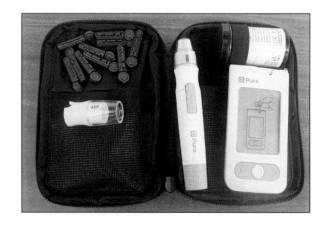

67 Insulin testing kit. Check airline security procedures ahead of time: some items may need to be labeled.

- Most people with diabetes obtain a license. Erratic control, hypoglycemia, and poor eyesight are the usual reasons for being refused a license.
- To avoid hypoglycemia patients should be educated as to the nature and treatment of hypoglycemia and should:
  - ◇ Check their blood glucose before driving.
  - ◇ Not drive for more than 2 hours.
  - ◇ Have glucose available in the car if needed.
  - ◇ Not delay a meal or snack.
  - ◇ Stop driving if there are any suggestions that they are developing hypoglycemic symptoms.
- Patients with diabetes should not drive if they have just started insulin, have erratic control, have difficulty with hypoglycemia, or have impaired vision not corrected with glasses.
- The American Diabetes Association has a useful set of tips aimed mainly at younger and recently qualified drivers, accessible at www.diabetes.org/living-with-diabetes/parents-and-kids/everyday-life/driving.html:
  - ◇ **Pass the test.** Check your blood glucose before getting into the car. Every time. No exceptions.
  - ◇ **Stop for a diabetes red light.** Treat low blood glucose and then recheck in 15 minutes. Do not get behind the wheel until blood glucose is in the target range.
  - ◇ **Slow down.** Treat blood glucose even if it means being late. It's never OK to drive with a low blood glucose. Call whoever is waiting for you and explain why you'll be a little late. They'll understand.
  - ◇ **Always have enough fuel.** Stock the car with healthy, nonperishable snacks and fast-acting sugars. And keep your diabetic supplies within easy reach.
  - ◇ **Pull over.** Pull over immediately if you are feeling sick or low while driving. Check your blood glucose, treat yourself, wait 15 minutes, and then recheck.
  - ◇ **ID, please.** Don't leave home without a driver's license and medical ID bracelet or necklace. Always wear medical ID.

Patients who have just started insulin, have erratic control, have difficulty with hypoglycemia, or have impaired vision not corrected with glasses should not drive.

Diabetes screening and patient care

CHAPTER 6

Diabetes and vascular disease

Macrovascular disease

◆ In industrialized countries, macrovascular disease is the major cause of mortality.

◆ The mortality rates for patients with type 2 diabetes, which varies between populations, are up to four times those of the nondiabetic population and this excess mortality has been attributed mainly to accelerated macrovascular disease, in particular cardiovascular disease (**68**).

◆ Diabetes remains the commonest single cause of limb amputations, as well as the commonest cause of blindness and renal failure in middle-aged adults in developed countries.

◆ Risk factors associated with a predisposition to macrovascular disease include diabetes and impaired glucose tolerance, hypertension, obesity, hypertriglyceridemia, and decreased HDL-cholesterol levels.

  ◇ These risk factors typically cluster in any one person, i.e. the prevalence of each factor is increased in those individuals with the other factors, leading to a self-perpetuating vicious cycle, which is further exaggerated in type 2 diabetes patients.

  ◇ These metabolic, hemodynamic, and constitutional changes do not represent a single disease but are considered to be a syndrome associated with hyperinsulinemia – metabolic or insulin-resistance syndrome (see p. 50).

  ◇ Such an insulin-resistant state may be present in 25% of the nondiabetic population, and about 2–12% per year of these individuals in adult life progress to diabetes.

◆ Since the metabolic or insulin-resistance syndrome represents a continuum into a state associated with major clinical consequences, there are three implications for the practicing physician in identifying this syndrome in any single patient:

  ◇ Identification of any one of the changes associated with the syndrome should lead to a search for other features of the syndrome.

  ◇ The approach to the management of a diabetic patient should not be viewed simply as the management of blood glucose.

  ◇ The management of each patient with type 2 diabetes must be tailored to the particular risk factor profile identified in that individual.

Mortality in adults with type 2 diabetes is far higher than in the nondiabetic population, largely because of cardiovascular disease.

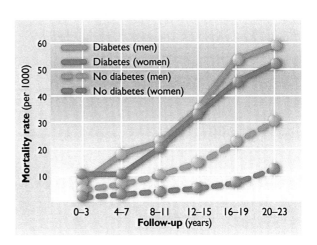

68 Cardiovascular risk. There is increasing risk with disease duration. Note also the relatively high risk in diabetic women, compared with nondiabetic women.

Pathogenesis of macrovascular complications

- Normal vascular homeostasis is regulated by an intricately interrelated network of endothelial and smooth muscle cells.
  - ◇ Endothelial cells act as a semipermeable gateway, which maintain the blood in a liquid state and produce mediators that promote vascular homeostasis (notably nitric oxide and lipid factors, such as prostacyclin).
  - ◇ Contraction of smooth muscle cells regulates the vascular tone of arteriolar walls, thereby determining both systolic blood pressure and peripheral blood flow.
- In diabetes, this intricate network is disturbed, resulting in atherogenesis. Endothelial cell dysfunction occurs early in the pathology of atherosclerosis and is common in patients with traditional risk factors – even in the absence of manifest atherosclerotic lesions. Such endothelial dysfunction predicts both progression to atherosclerosis and major cardiovascular events, such as myocardial infarction.
- The pathogenesis of atherosclerosis, from the initial phase of leukocyte recruitment to late events, such as rupture of vulnerable plaques, predominantly involves inflammatory processes, including the release of inflammatory mediators (**69**). This leads to an elevation of several inflammatory markers in the peripheral blood of patients with atherosclerosis, as well as patients with type 2 diabetes.
  - ◇ An example is C-reactive protein (CRP), which is an acute-phase reactant thought to be a marker of vascular inflammation. CRP is localized within the atheromatous plaque and its expression precedes the recruitment of leukocytes at the surface of the vessel wall. Since levels of CRP and other proinflammatory mediators, such as fibrinogen, are increased in the plasma of patients with diabetes they may serve as clinical biomarkers of vascular risk.
- The pathogenesis of atherosclerosis in diabetes is as in nondiabetic subjects, but with the added burden of hyperglycemia and its impact on cell function, allied to the clustering of other risk factors found in the metabolic syndrome.

69 Atherosclerosis. Damage to arterial endothelium allows entry of monocytes and lipids (1) and activation of macrophages (2). The macrophages engulf the lipids, subsequently breaking down into foam cells and causing lipid accumulation on the vessel wall (3, 4). The release of cytokines stimulates migration of smooth muscle cells to form a fibrous cap (5, 6).

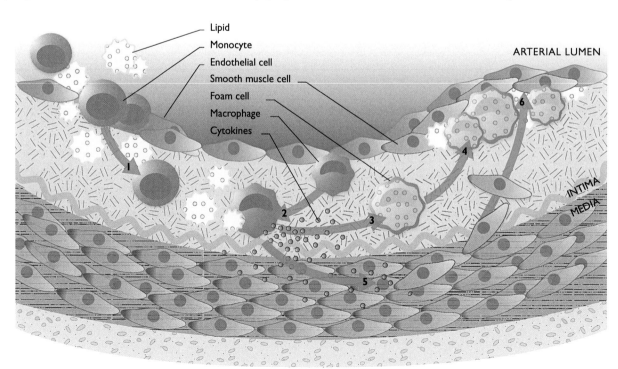

Lipid
Monocyte
Endothelial cell
Smooth muscle cell
Foam cell
Macrophage
Cytokines

ARTERIAL LUMEN

INTIMA
MEDIA

Treatment and management principles for macrovascular disease

General principles

◆ In the diabetic patient with macrovascular disease, management is directed at correcting symptoms, reducing mortality risk, and treating the anatomical lesion.

◆ To correct symptoms, consider drugs to reduce angina, including nitrates, beta-adrenoreceptor blockers, long-acting calcium channel blockers, and potassium channel openers.

◆ To reduce mortality risk, consider drugs to limit cardiovascular disease progression, including aspirin, statins, and angiotensin-converting enzyme inhibitors (ACEIs).

◇ Use statins and aspirin in all diabetic patients with macrovascular disease, plus fibrates to correct hypertriglyceridemia and increase HDL as necessary.

◇ Fibrates must be used cautiously in patients taking statins because of the risk of rhabdo-myolysis.

◇ If statins and fibrates have to be used concur-rently, fenofibrate is recommended over gemfibrozil, as gemfibrozil interferes with statin glucuronidation, thereby conferring a higher risk of myopathy and rhabdomyolysis than does fenofibrate.

◆ To reduce mortality risk there is also the need to achieve tight glycemic control.

◆ To correct the anatomical lesions, consider surgical intervention to improve revasculariza-tion, in order to control symptoms and improve prognosis. There are two techniques for success-ful cardiac revascularization:

◇ Percutaneous intervention.

◇ Coronary bypass surgery.

◆ The role of cerebrovascular revascularization remains unclear in diabetes and it should be used as for nondiabetic patients.

Strict glycemic control significantly improves the prognosis in the diabetic patient with a myocardial infarction.

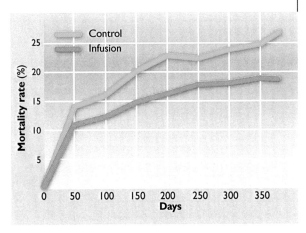

70 Glycemic control and cardiovascular outcomes. The DIGAMI study demonstrated decreased mortality in patients receiving insulin–glucose infusion against control patients over the course of 1 year.

Glucose control

◆ Patients with hyperglycemia on admission for a myocardial infarction have a poorer prognosis than patients with normoglycemia.

◆ The rise in creatine kinase (CK)-MB enzymes, which reflects the extent of cardiac muscle infarc-tion, is greater in patients with elevated blood glucose concentrations.

◆ In patients presenting with an acute myocardial infarction, the Diabetes Mellitus Insulin Glucose Infusion in Acute Myocardial Infarction (DIGAMI) study showed that strict glycemic control in the diabetic patient significantly improved cardio-vascular outcomes (**70**).

◇ This study used an insulin–glucose infusion for about 24 hours followed by multiple sub-cutaneous insulin dosing for 3 months. DIGAMI-2 tried to discover whether it was the insulin–glucose infusion, the sub-cutaneous insulin, or both that led to the improvement; however, difficulties in carrying out the study resulted in all three groups achieving similar glucose control.

◇ The question of acute versus subsequent tight control was not answered by this study, but the overall excellent HbA1c achieved at the end of the study (~6.8% [51 mmol/mol] for all groups) was associated with improved cardiovascular outcomes in all groups. A 2% increase in HbA1c was associated with a 20% increase in mortality.

Diabetes and vascular disease

In light of other studies showing improved morbidity and mortality in critically ill patients, it is recommended that patients with diabetes presenting with an acute coronary syndrome or myocardial infarction be treated with insulin infusions to maintain blood glucose control at 5–8.2 mmol/l (90–145 mg/dl) as per guidelines (e.g. American Heart Association).

Lipid-lowering drugs

The Long-Term Intervention with Pravastatin in Ischemic Disease (LIPID) trial showed that in patients with diabetes or impaired fasting glucose, with a previous myocardial infarction or unstable angina and total plasma cholesterol level of 4.0–7.0 mmol/l (154–270 mg/dl), pravastatin reduced the incidence of cardiovascular events, including stroke.

In the Cholesterol and Recurrent Events (CARE) trial, pravastatin was given to adults with myocardial infarction, total cholesterol levels less than 6.2 mmol/l (240 mg/dl) and LDL-cholesterol levels of 3.0–4.5 mmol/l (115–174 mg/dl). The primary endpoint – of fatal coronary event or a nonfatal myocardial infarction – was significantly reduced with pravastatin compared to placebo. This reduction was seen in both diabetic and nondiabetic patients.

With regard to fibrates, the Veterans Affairs HDL Intervention Trial (VA-HIT) showed that gemfibrozil reduced the incidence of myocardial infarction and stroke in patients, including diabetes patients, with coronary artery disease plus low HDL- and high LDL-cholesterol levels.

Revascularization procedures

Coronary revascularization relieves symptoms and, in certain subgroups, particularly patients with advanced three-vessel or left main stem disease, improves prognosis.

Thresholds for angiography should be low in diabetes.

◇ This is not only because of diabetes patients' heightened risk and poorer outlook, but also because symptoms are often atypical, perhaps because of abnormalities in the perception of angina caused by autonomic neuropathy (**71**).

Revascularization procedures in diabetes may be technically demanding and potentially hazardous because the diffuse and severe arterial disease makes clear targets for stenting or graft insertion hard to identify.

The Bypass Angioplasty Revascularization Investigation (BARI) Trial showed that coronary artery bypass grafting (CABG) resulted in a lower cardiac mortality than percutaneous transluminal coronary angioplasty (PTCA) in diabetic patients.

However, the introduction of stenting plus the more potent antithrombotic agents, particularly glycoprotein IIb/IIIa receptor blockers, has improved prognosis.

◇ In the Evaluation of PTCA to Improve Long-term Outcome by c7E3 GP IIb/IIIa Receptor Blockade (EPILOG) Trial, abciximab (a platelet aggregation inhibitor) given during PTCA was associated with a significant reduction in death or myocardial infarction in both diabetic and nondiabetic patients.

◇ In a predefined subgroup analysis from the Evaluation of Platelet IIb/IIIa Inhibitor for Stenting (EPISTENT) trial showed that stenting combined with infusion of abciximab improved the long-term outcome in diabetic patients substantially. In a combined analysis the 1-year incidence of ischemic endpoints was comparable to that achieved in nondiabetic patients.

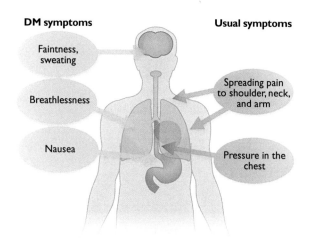

DM symptoms

Faintness, sweating

Breathlessness

Nausea

Usual symptoms

Spreading pain to shoulder, neck, and arm

Pressure in the chest

71 Symptoms of angina. Diabetic patients may exhibit atypical symptoms, such as weakness, faintness, sweating, nausea, and breathing difficulty, as well as a reduced pain sensitivity.

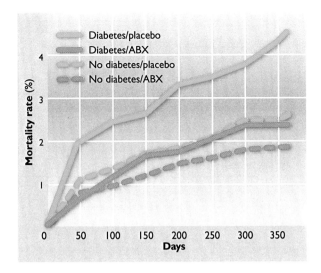

72 Abciximab therapy and PTCA. Combined data from the three placebo-controlled trials, EPISTENT, EPILOG, and EPIC, showed that abciximab (ABX) substantially decreased the mortality of diabetic patients. *Adapted from Bhatt DL et al.*

◇ The results of the EPILOG, EPISTENT, and one other study on abciximab, the Evaluation of Platelet IIb/IIIa Inhibition for Prevention of Ischemic Complications (EPIC) trial, were pooled. The combined analysis showed that abciximab reduced the mortality of diabetic patients to the level of nondiabetic patients receiving placebo (**72**).

Factors associated with the pathogenesis of microvascular complications

Hyperglycemia
Protein glycation
Advanced glycation endproducts (AGE)
Reactive oxygen species (ROS)
Activation of cell NFκB
Sorbitol accumulation in cells
Activation of cell protein kinase C
Hemodynamic changes

Microvascular disease

◆ Whereas macrovascular disease affects both diabetic and nondiabetic people, microvascular disease is only seen in people with diabetes, and a few other conditions such as hypertension.
◆ Small blood vessels throughout the body are affected but the disease process has a particular clinical impact at three sites:
  ◇ Retina (retinopathy).
  ◇ Renal glomerulus (nephropathy).
  ◇ Nerve sheaths (neuropathy).

Pathogenesis of microvascular complications

◆ The cause of diabetic microvascular disease is not known, but several factors are understood to play a role (**73**).
◆ In some ways the factors causing this form of vascular disease are similar to those involved in macrovascular disease, for example:
  ◇ Hypertension is a risk factor in microvascular renal and eye disease.
  ◇ Smoking is a risk factor in renal disease.
◆ Hyperglycemia is not a major factor in macrovascular disease, but is critical in the development of microvascular disease. Hypertension is just as important in predisposing to microvascular disease as hyperglycemia and all the five modifiable factors targeted by therapy are relevant:
  ◇ Hyperglycemia.
  ◇ Hypertension.
  ◇ Hyperlipidemia.
  ◇ Lack of exercise.
  ◇ Smoking.

Hyperglycemia is critical in the development of microvascular disease.

---

73 Causes of microvascular disease. There is a direct causal link between hyperglycemia and microangiopathy, although there are several other contributing factors.

74 **Pathogenesis of diabetic microangiopathy.** Excess glucose causes an array of abnormalities, eventually leading to basement membrane thickening, endothelial cell changes, and pericyte cell death.

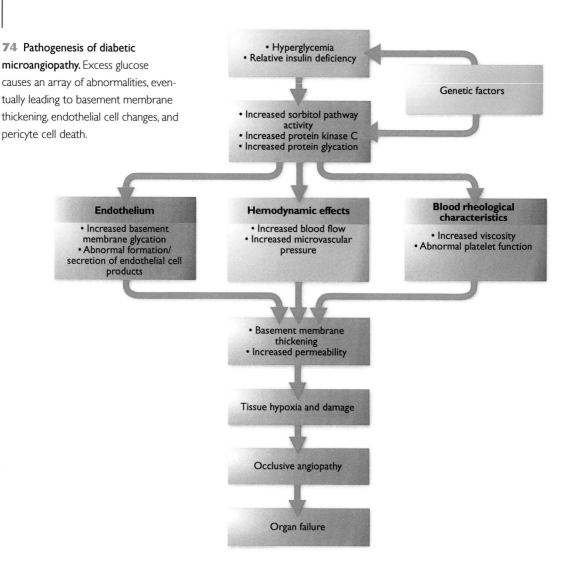

While hyperglycemia is the primary metabolic dysfunction in microvascular complications, the main target is the endothelial cell (**74**).

Hyperglycemia

Hyperglycemia predisposes to diabetic microvascular disease; reducing hyperglycemia can limit that progression and prevent disease development, as illustrated by DCCT for type 1 diabetes and UKPDS for type 2 diabetes:

◇ In terms of reducing risk for microvascular complications, the DCCT showed that intensive glycemic control in type 1 diabetes reduced the risk of developing retinopathy in the primary prevention cohort (no retinopathy at baseline) by 76%, microalbuminuria by 34%, and neuropathy by 71% compared to conventional treatment.

◇ In the UKPDS study of newly diagnosed type 2 diabetic patients, intensive glycemic control was associated with a reduced risk of microvascular endpoints, including microalbuminuria retinopathy.

◇ In the Kumamoto study on thin type 2 diabetic Japanese patients, those in the intensive glycemic treatment group had a 76% risk reduction for retinopathy and 57% for microalbuminuria in the primary prevention cohort.

There are several possible mechanisms linking hyperglycemia and diabetic microvascular disease (**75**).

75 Oxidative stress pathways. Hyperglycemia leads to oxidative stress and diabetic complications via several seemingly independent mechanisms: polyol pathway activation, advanced glycation endproduct (AGE) formation, protein kinase C (PKC) activation, and hexosamine pathway activation.

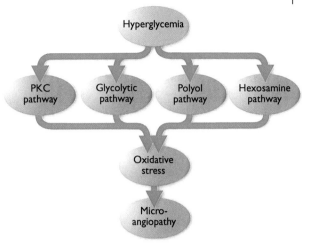

High intracellular glucose

◆ When glucose is high inside a cell, most of it is metabolized by glycolysis, first to glucose-6-phosphate, then to fructose-6-phosphate, and on through the glycolytic pathway. Some fructose-6-phosphate is diverted into the hexosamine pathway in which it is converted to N-acetyl glucosamine, which can modify gene expression.

◆ At the same time, high intracellular glucose causes increased mitochondrial production of reactive oxygen species (ROS). ROS can cause strand breaks in nuclear DNA, which can reduce the activity of key enzymes and activate less beneficial pathways.

◆ Broadly, the consequence of high intracellular glucose is that the cell is stressed and mounts an anti-stress response to try to restore homeostasis.

76 AGE reactions. The interaction of advanced glycation endproducts (AGE) with arterial wall components increases vascular permeability and wall thickness, the expression of pro-coagulant activity, the generation of reactive oxygen species (ROS), and the endothelial expression of adhesion molecules. NFκB, a transcription factor; IGF-1, insulin-like growth factor 1; VEGF, vascular endothelial growth factor; VCAM-1, vascular cell adhesion molecule-1.

Advanced glycation endproducts

◆ Long-term modification of proteins by protein glycation and oxidation leads to the formation of advanced glycation endproducts (AGE) (**76**). AGE precursors damage cells via:

◇ Modification of intracellular proteins, including proteins involved in regulation of gene transcription.

◇ Modification of extracellular matrix molecules on diffusion out of cells, which alters matrix–cell signaling and causes cellular dysfunction.

◇ Modification of circulating blood proteins which bind to AGE receptors and activate them, causing inflammation and vascular pathology.

◆ Tissue levels of AGE increase with age, and can be derived from exogenous sources such as food and tobacco smoke.

Diabetes and vascular disease

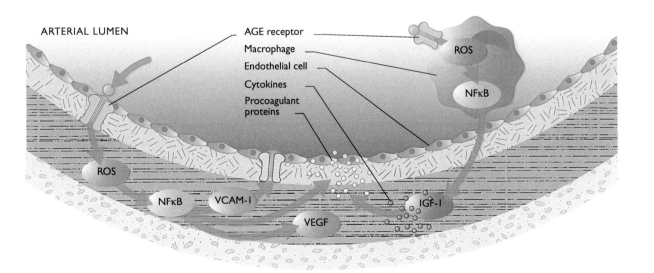

Reactive oxygen species

◆ Increased production of ROS causes reduced availability of nitric oxide, with loss of its anti-inflammatory, anti-proliferative, and anti-adhesive properties.

◆ *Activation of NFκB:* this critical complex involved in cellular immune responses can be activated by oxidative stress and binding of AGEs to cell receptors on inflammatory cells including macrophages. AGE engagement with these AGE receptors (RAGE) promotes expression of pro-inflammatory cytokines, procoagulants and vaso-constriction.

Sorbitol accumulation

◆ Aldose reductase normally reduces toxic aldehydes in the cell to inactive alcohols, but when the glucose concentration in the cell is high, aldose reductase also reduces that glucose to sorbitol, which is later oxidized to fructose (**77**).

◆ In the process of reducing high intracellular glucose to sorbitol, the aldose reductase consumes the cofactor NADPH. NADPH is also the essential cofactor for regenerating a critical intracellular antioxidant, reduced glutathione.

◆ By decreasing reduced glutathione, the polyol pathway increases susceptibility to intracellular oxidative stress.

◆ As a result, there is a cellular 'pseudohypoxia' as well as accumulation of the osmotically active sorbitol. Sorbitol can damage these cells.

◆ Aldose reductase inhibitors limit sorbitol formation.

Activation of protein kinase C-beta

◆ High glucose inside a cell increases the synthesis of diacylglycerol, which is a critical activating cofactor for protein kinase C-beta (PKC-β), an enzyme which regulates vascular permeability, contractility, and proliferation.

◆ PKC-β activation by high intracellular glucose influences gene expression pathologically. For example, the vasodilator producing endothelial nitric oxide synthase (eNOS) is decreased, while the vasoconstrictor endothelin-1, implicated in diabetic eye disease, is increased.

---

*Glucose + NADPH + H+ leads to
(aldose reductase) Sorbitol + NADP+.*

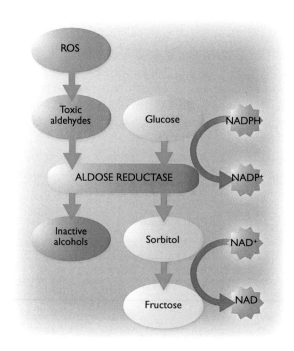

77 Sorbitol conversion. Aldose reductase reduces toxic aldehydes generated by ROS to inactive alcohols, and excess glucose to sorbitol, subsequently oxidizing the sorbitol to fructose, and using NADPH and NAD+ as co-factors. However, this consumption of NADPH can lead to decreased glutathione reductase and further oxidative stress.

Hemodynamic changes

◆ In diabetes there is increased blood viscosity and shear stress, with plugging of capillaries by activated leukocytes, as well as chronic hypoxia due to closure and nonperfusion of capillaries with proliferation of new vessels.

◆ Activation of pro-adhesive mechanisms in retino-pathy can cause white cells to plug capillaries with consequent problems with perfusion. New vessels grow to bring blood back to the periphery, but these new vessels are inadequate at revascularizing ischemic areas, grow from the venous side of the retinal circulation, bleed easily, and cause the growth of fibrous tissue.

Treatment and management principles for microvascular disease

◆ Microvascular disease is influenced by several modifiable factors, including hyperglycemia, hypertension, dyslipidemia, and smoking.

◆ Microvascular disease is also influenced by several unmodifiable factors, including:

◇ *Duration of diabetes.* Complications tend to manifest themselves 10–20 years after diagnosis in young patients. A patient who does not develop renal disease by 30 years postdiagnosis is unlikely to develop that complication. Retinopathy can be present at diagnosis of type 2 diabetes, probably because the patient had unrecognized diabetes for several years prior to diagnosis.

◇ *Genetic factors.* Diabetic siblings of diabetic patients with renal and eye disease have a 3–5-fold increased risk of the same complication compared to siblings of patients without renal or eye disease. Patients with diabetes due to a glucokinase polymorphism associated with raised fasting glucose but minimal postprandial hyperglycemia rarely develop microvascular complications.

◇ *Racial factors.* Some races are at higher risk of microvascular complications than others. For example, in the US, the rank order of risk is Pima American Indians > Hispanic/Mexican origin > US African origin > US European origin patients.

Reducing the risk of vascular disease

◆ In the diabetic patient without vascular disease, management is directed at reducing risk for these complications, primarily by addressing a set of modifiable risk factors (**78**).

◆ Prevention of microvascular complications reduces morbidity in diabetic patients, while reduction of cardiovascular risk is of prime importance, since this is the major contributor to both mortality and morbidity.

◇ The Multiple Risk Factor Intervention Trial (MRFIT) showed increasing likelihood of death from cardiovascular disease, according to the number of risk factors present (**79**).

78 Risk factors in vascular disease. Risk factors can be either modifiable by therapy or life-style changes, or – as with age or gender – not modifiable.

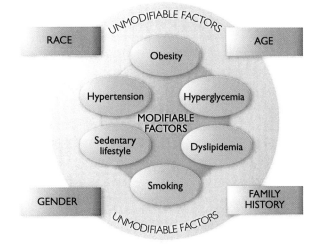

79 Cardiovascular risk. Among the 347,978 men aged 35–57 years, screened for inclusion in the MRFIT trial, were 5163 who reported taking medication for diabetes. In both diabetic and nondiabetic men, the number of risk factors (dyslipidemia, hypertension, or smoking) independently predicted cardiovascular disease (CVD) mortality, with the diabetic patients having a higher CVD death rate than nondiabetics with one or even two other cardiovascular risk factors.

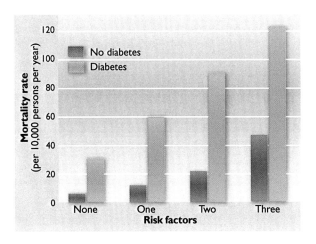

Diabetes and vascular disease

Obesity and sedentary lifestyle

◆ Central to the prevention of cardiovascular disease is behavior modification (**80**).

◆ Diet and exercise are always advocated, though their importance has been cast aside by many patients because of the difficulty in achieving the goals – as compared with the relative ease of taking pills, or doing nothing – to address hypertension and dyslipidemia.

◆ Dietary recommendations include limiting saturated fat to <7% of total caloric intake, having two or more servings of fish per week to provide polyunsaturated fatty acids, and incorporating fruits, vegetables, legumes, low-fat dairy products, and whole grains into meals.

◆ Aim for 150 minutes per week of moderate intensity aerobic physical activity (50–70% maximum heart rate); in the absence of contraindications, people with type 2 diabetes should be encouraged to perform resistance training three times per week. (American Diabetes Association [ADA] guidelines).

Hypertension

◆ The UKPDS trial concluded that tight blood pressure (BP) control in patients with hypertension and type 2 diabetes achieves a clinically important reduction in the risk of diabetes-related deaths and complications.

◆ The initial therapy for borderline hypertension in diabetes patients (within 10 mmHg of the target pressure) is exercise (30 minutes brisk walking per day) and sodium restriction (<100 mmol or <2.3 g per day). Weight loss also improves BP, partly by reducing insulin resistance.

◆ If the BP target – which varies with a number of factors including age and recommending agency – has not been reached with these nonpharmacological measures, thiazide diuretics, angiotensin-converting-enzyme inhibitors (ACEIs), angiotensin-receptor blockers (ARBs), beta-blockers, and/or calcium-channel blockers should be employed.

◆ Particular care should be taken when initiating therapy in patients aged above 70 years, or if there is postural hypotension, hypovolemia, or renal impairment.

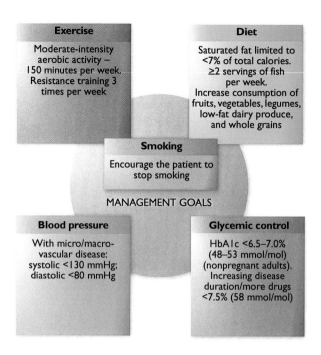

80 Prevention and management. A combination of behavior modification and tight glycemic and blood pressure control can significantly reduce cardiovascular risk.

◆ UK NICE guidelines recommend ACEIs in general, but for Afro-Caribbean patients ACEIs plus either a diuretic or calcium-channel blocker. These three agents are first- and second-line therapy and can then be used in any combination to achieve the target.

◆ Multiple studies, such as the Hypertension Optimal Treatment (HOT) trial, UKPDS, and the Anti-Hypertensive and Lipid-Lowering Treatment to Prevent Heart Attacks Trials (ALLHAT), have shown that two or more antihypertensive agents are usually needed.

◆ For most patients, ACEIs are the initial treatment of choice, assuming the patient can tolerate them. The second drug of choice is either a calcium-channel blocker (based on the ASCOT study) for a patient without nephropathy, or a thiazide diuretic (based on the ALLHAT).

◇ Women who are pregnant or might become pregnant should avoid ACEI and ARB drugs and start with calcium-channel blockers.

◆ In the ALLHAT, there was no significant difference in the risk of fatal coronary heart disease and nonfatal myocardial infarction between a thiazide, ACEI, and calcium-channel blocker.

- An ACEI reduced the risk of microalbuminuria in type 2 diabetes patients with hypertension and normoalbuminuria in the Bergamo Nephrologic Diabetes Complications Trial (BENEDICT), so it can be argued that the renoprotective effect makes ACEIs the first choice.
- ACEIs are also debatably the initial drug of choice, based on a cardioprotective effect, in patients aged over 55 years with type 2 diabetes and a cardiovascular risk of at least 20% in the next 10 years.
- The Micro-HOPE study demonstrated decreasing risk of major vascular events with ramipril in diabetes patients with a previous cardiovascular event.
  - ◇ 577 people with diabetes aged 55 years or older, with a previous cardiovascular event or at least one other cardiovascular risk factor, were randomly assigned ramipril (10 mg/day) or placebo. The study was stopped after 4.5 years.
  - ◇ Ramipril lowered the risk of the combined primary outcome by 25%, myocardial infarction by 22%, stroke by 33%, total mortality by 24%, and overt nephropathy by 24%. The cardiovascular benefit of ramipril was greater than that attributable to the decrease in blood pressure.

- If ACEIs are indicated but not tolerated, then ARBs should be considered.
  - ◇ The commonest reason for withdrawing an ACEI is a chronic dry cough, which reflects angioedema of the bronchus.
- With either ACEIs or ARBs, it is recommended that serum potassium and creatinine be checked 1 week after starting since hyperkalemia and further renal dysfunction can ensue if concomitant renal artery stenosis is present.
- Beta-adrenergic blockers and alpha-adrenergic blockers are useful as add-on medications to control BP, though the adverse metabolic risk with hyperglycemia and dyslipidemia favors the latter and adrenergic blockers are now relegated in the list of options below calcium-channel blocking agents and thiazides (**81**). Potassium-sparing diuretics can also be used at this stage.
- Short-acting calcium-channel blockers should be avoided.

81 Drug therapy for hypertension. Of the six main classes of antihypertension drugs used in diabetes ACEIs are the drug of choice, partly because they tend to give the greatest BP reduction and improved cardiovascular outcomes. However, there is substantial variation among individuals.

Diabetes and vascular disease

Antihypertensive agents for type 2 diabetes

DRUG CLASS	ADVANTAGES	DISADVANTAGES
ACEIs	Reduce microalbuminuria Improve cardiovascular outcomes Beneficial in heart failure	Can cause hyperkalemia Can worsen renal function if with renal artery stenosis
Thiazide diuretics	Inexpensive	Can cause hypokalemia Usually not effective when serum creatinine reaches 159.1 μmol/l (1.8 mg/dl)
ARBs	Decrease risk of progression of micro-albuminuria and later stages of nephropathy	Can cause hyperkalemia Can worsen renal function if with renal artery stenosis
Beta-blockers	Reduce cardiovascular outcomes especially postmyocardial infarction	Hyperglycemia and dyslipidemia Can reduce adrenergic symptoms accompanying hypoglycemia
Calcium-channel blockers	Effective	Can cause peripheral edema
Alpha-blockers	Effective	Can cause postural hypotension

Dyslipidemia

◆ Different therapies are available depending on the nature of the dyslipidemia (**82**).

◆ The Collaborative Atorvastatin Diabetes Study (CARDS) showed that statins can reduce the risk of a first cardiovascular event (**83**).

◇ In type 2 diabetic patients who had no previous history of cardiovascular disease but with either hypertension, albuminuria, retinopathy, or were currently smoking, atorvastatin 10 mg daily resulted in primary prevention of acute coronary events and stroke. Mean LDL-cholesterol at entry was 3.04 mmol/l (117.4 mg/dl) for the atorvastatin group and 3.02 mmol/l (116.6 mg/dl) for the placebo group; and at the end of the study these were 2.11 mmol/l (81.5 mg/dl) and 3.12 mmol/l (120.5 mg/dl) respectively.

◆ Statins and aspirin are currently recommended:

◇ Either simplistically for all diabetes patients aged 40 years or more.

◇ Or for patients with LDL-C >2.5 mmol/l or 100 mg/dl.

◇ Or, using a personalized approach, for those diabetes patients with a 20% 10-year risk of progression to macrovascular disease.

◆ High doses of statins have a greater benefit than low doses in the absence of side-effects so treatment with simvastatin 40 mg or atorvastatin 20 mg is often recommended, even when the lipid target has been achieved with a lower dose.

Pharmacological management of adverse lipid profile

LIPID ABNORMALITY	DRUG
Elevated LDL-cholesterol	Statins Ezetimibe Niacin Bile acid sequestrants
Elevated triglycerides	Fibrates Fish oils Ezetimibe Niacin
Low HDL-cholesterol	Niacin Fibrates

82 Dyslipidemia therapies. Different drugs are used for different lipid abnormalities.

◆ Fibrates to correct hypertriglyceridemia and increase HDL are also suggested, though recent trials suggest that niacin may be preferable to fenofibrate for hypertriglyceridemia.

◇ The Fenofibrate Intervention and Event Lowering in Diabetes (FIELD) study found that fenofibrate therapy reduced lower-limb amputation events in patients with type 2 diabetes (**84**).

◆ Fibrates must be used cautiously in patients taking statins because of the risk of rhabdomyolysis.

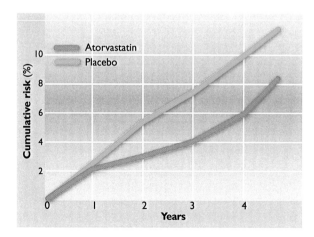

83 Effect of statins. Diabetes patients taking atorvastatin demonstrated reduced cardiovascular and mortality risk. *Adapted from the CARDS study: Colhoun H et al.*

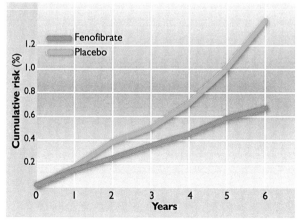

84 Effect of fibrates. Fenofibrate lowered the long-term risk of minor amputations for diabetes patients. *Adapted from the FIELD study: Rajamani K et al.*

- If statins and fibrates have to be used concurrently, fenofibrate is recommended over gemfibrozil because of a lower risk of myopathy and rhabdomyolysis. This greater risk is because gemfibrozil interferes with statin glucuronidation.
- Other medications such as ezetimibe, niacin, and bile acid sequestrants play a role when desired lipid levels are not achieved with statins and fibrates.
- The mode of action of statins, fibrates, and other lipid-lowering drugs is shown in **85**.

Smoking

- Stopping smoking reduces the risk of cardiovascular disease by up to 70% in nondiabetic subjects and the same is probably true in patients with diabetes.
- All patients of any age should be advised against smoking. This is especially true in children who are at greatest risk of starting to smoke.
- At the annual review smoking habits should be documented and patients encouraged to stop or reduce the numbers of cigarettes.
- Counseling in combination with nicotine supplements is more effective at reducing smoking than nicotine supplements alone.
- Buproprion or varenicline are alternative therapies to stop smoking but should be prescribed for short periods, in combination with counseling, and with strict adherence to guidelines, such as avoiding their use in depression.

Hyperglycemia

- Glycemic control can be assessed by measuring the average blood glucose levels with glycated (or glycosylated) hemoglobin (HbA1/HbA1c).
  - ◇ Glycation of hemoglobin occurs as a non-enzymatic two-step reaction, resulting in the formation of a covalent bond between the glucose molecule and the terminal valine of the beta chain of the hemoglobin molecule.
  - ◇ The percentage of hemoglobin glycated is related to the prevailing glucose concentration, intracellular glucose metabolism, and the lifespan of the red cell.
  - ◇ Glycated hemoglobin is expressed as a percentage of the normal hemoglobin (normal range approximately 4–8% [DCCT] or 20–64 mmol/mol [IFCC] depending on the technique of measurement).

85 Lipid-lowering drugs. Very-low-density lipoproteins (VLDL) are precursors of cholesterol-rich, atherogenic LDL. Some drugs target the metabolism of VLDL by affecting apolipoprotein expression, some improve the clearance of LDL from the circulation, and others increase HDL production.

Statins

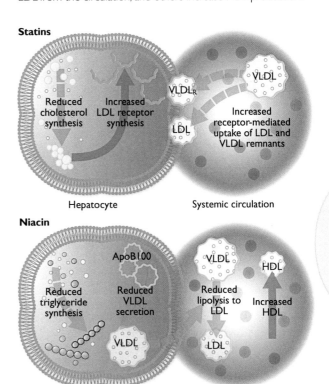

Niacin

Fibrates

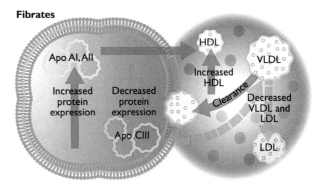

Ezetimibe

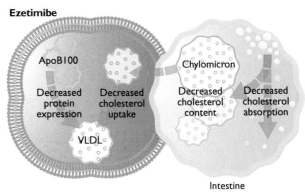

Diabetes and vascular disease

◇ HbA1c provides an index of the average blood glucose concentration over the life of the hemoglobin molecule (over a 6–12-week period). The level of HbA1c provides an index of hyperglycemia, and thus diabetes control, over that period.

◇ The figure will be misleading if the lifespan of the red cell changes, either due to altered red cell survival, as in renal failure, or an abnormal hemoglobin, as in thalassemia.

◆ Recently, HbA1c estimations have been standardized and the improved accuracy, allied to the poor reproducibility of oral glucose tolerance tests, has led to suggestions that HbA1c could be used as a screening test to alert physicians to the possibility of diabetes.

◇ In broad terms, HbA1c levels >6.5% (48 mmol/mol) are associated with a risk of diabetic microvascular disease (retinopathy), while lower levels, even into the normal range, are associated with an increased risk of macrovascular disease.

◇ ADA guidelines aim for HbA1c <7.0% (53 mmol/mol) (nonpregnant adults). UK NICE guidelines aim for HbA1c <6.5% (48 mmol/mol) initially; later with increasing disease duration and more drugs aim less low, i.e. <7.5% (58 mmol/mol).

◆ Glycated plasma proteins (fructosamine) can also be measured as an index of control and relate to a shorter period of diabetes control (2–3 weeks).

◇ This can be of value in patients with a hemoglobinopathy or in pregnancy (when hemoglobin turnover is changeable) and other situations that require rapid changes of treatment.

◆ Strict glycemic control did not reduce macrovascular complications in the UKPDS by a statistically significant degree in the first 15 years, but did so thereafter.

◇ A recent finding in type 1 diabetic patients followed from the original DCCT showed that tight glycemic control resulted in less cardiovascular disease (i.e. nonfatal myocardial infarction, stroke, death from cardiovascular disease, confirmed angina, or the need for coronary artery revascularization), compared to conventional treatment.

◆ By contrast, tight glycemic control has a marked effect on the onset of microvascular complications (see p. 78) in both type 1 and type 2 diabetes patients. However, only 11% of the variation in microvascular complication risk is attributable to HbA1c change.

◆ In the UK, NICE recommends the initiation of therapy with lifestyle intervention and then with metformin. Should the HbA1c rise above 6.5% (48 mmol/mol) then a sulfonylurea or a glinide may be prescribed (for those with a nonroutine lifestyle). NICE recommend considering a thiazolidinedione (TZD) if the side-effects of sulfonylureas are unacceptable.

◇ Should the HbA1c rise above 7.5% (58 mmol/mol) then NICE recommend the addition of TZDs or insulin or exenatide (if weight is a particular problem).

◆ The stepwise increase in drug therapy is a topic of debate in academic circles, while the lack of mention of DPP-4 inhibitors or the GLP-1 analog liraglutide (as an alternative to exenatide) reflects the inevitable delay in producing guidelines that include current agents.

◇ Exenatide has now been studied for use in combination with insulin glargine, and liraglutide with insulin glargine and insulin detemir.

Antithrombotic agents

◆ Statins and aspirin are currently recommended for all diabetes patients aged >40 years; some physicians prefer to individualize cardiovascular disease risk, starting statins when this is in excess of 20% over 10 years.

◆ Following recent studies, the case for aspirin in those under 65 years of age without cardiovascular disease is much less clear. The UK NICE guidelines point out that aspirin is not licensed for primary prevention treatment.

◆ The balance of benefit must be set against the risk of hemorrhage when on aspirin, and both will vary for different individuals with diabetes.

Diabetic neuropathy

Prevalence and classification

◆ Diabetic neuropathy is the most common complication of diabetes, conferring high morbidity.

◆ It is thought to be the result of several interrelated factors. Vascular abnormalities have been implicated in acute neuropathies, but without categorical evidence.

◆ It is difficult to estimate the prevalence of diabetic neuropathy, as it has a variety of manifestations and there are multiple diagnostic criteria; it varies from 20% of diabetic patients in simple clinical tests, such as perception of vibration, to >80% with more formal testing.

◆ Because of the variety in its presentation, several classification schemes are used to describe neuropathy (**86**), such as the following:

◇ Chronic sensory nerve disorders, which are usually distal symmetrical polyneuropathies and are the most common presentations of diabetic neuropathy.

◇ Acute sensory nerve disorders, which are usually asymmetrical, transient mononeuropathies.

◇ Acute motor neuropathies, which are uncommon.

◇ Autonomic neuropathy; the most common clinical manifestation is erectile dysfunction.

◆ An alternative classification scheme is to describe the neuropathy as diffuse (distal symmetric sensorimotor polyneuropathy, autonomic neuropathy) or focal (mononeuropathy, mononeuropathy multiplex, plexopathy, radiculopathy, cranial neuropathy).

Summary of diabetic neuropathy

SENSORIMOTOR NEUROPATHY

Distal symmetric polyneuropathy

Focal neuropathy
   Diabetic mononeuropathy
   (cranial, truncal, peripheral nerves)
   Mononeuropathy multiplex

Diabetic amyotrophy

AUTONOMIC NEUROPATHY

Hypoglycemic unawareness

Abnormal pupillary function

Cardiovascular autonomic neuropathy

Vasomotor neuropathy

Sudomotor neuropathy (sweat glands)

Gastrointestinal autonomic neuropathy
   Gastric atony
   Diabetic diarrhea or constipation
   Fecal incontinence

Genitourinary autonomic neuropathy
   Bladder dysfunction
   Sexual dysfunction

86 Classification of neuropathy. This scheme classifies sensory neuropathies as distal symmetric polyneuropathy, focal neuropathy, and diabetic amyotrophy. Autonomic neuropathies may be classified by the affected system, with motor neuropathies classified by the muscles that are involved.

Diagnosis

◆ The earliest functional change in diabetic nerves is delayed nerve conduction velocity.

◆ The earliest histological change is segmental demyelination caused by damage to Schwann cells. In the early stages, axons are preserved, implying prospects of recovery, but at a later stage irreversible axonal degeneration develops.

◆ The diagnosis of neuropathy can be made with such modalities as nerve conduction velocity and electromyography.

◆ In the outpatient setting, simpler tools are needed to diagnose diabetic neuropathy. Several neuro-pathy screening instruments, which involve scorecards grading physical exam findings (such as the presence or absence of ankle reflexes or vibration perception) have been developed, and vary in ease of use (**87**).

◆ The Semmes–Weinstein 5.07 (10 gram) mono-filament has been widely accepted as a screening tool for diabetic neuropathy (**88**).

◇ The monofilament is applied perpendicularly to nine sites on the plantar surface and one on the dorsal surface of the foot, with enough force to cause it to buckle; a variation is to apply it at only two sites – the plantar aspect of the first and fifth metatarsal heads (**89**).

◇ If the patient is unable to feel the mono-filament at these locations, this has 80% sensitivity and 86% specificity for diagnosing diabetic neuropathy.

87 Screening instruments. An example scorecard for staging diabetic foot disorders in order to assess the level of severity and the risk of problems. *Adapted from Feldman EL. Diabetes Care, 1994.*

Diabetic foot risk assessment chart

FEET (appearance)	RIGHT	LEFT
	Normal ☐	Normal ☐
	Abnormal (1) ☐	Abnormal (1) ☐
	Deformed (1) ☐	Deformed (1) ☐
	Dry skin, callus (1) ☐	Dry skin, callus (1) ☐
	Infection, fissure (1) ☐	Infection, fissure (1) ☐
ULCER		
	Absent ☐	Absent ☐
	Present (1) ☐	Present (1) ☐
ANKLE REFLEXES		
	Present ☐	Present ☐
	Present/reinforcement (0.5) ☐	Present (0.5) ☐
	Absent (1) ☐	Absent (1) ☐
VIBRATION (detected at first toe)		
	Present ☐	Present ☐
	Reduced (0.5) ☐	Reduced (0.5) ☐
	Absent (1) ☐	Absent (1) ☐
Total	☐ /8	☐ /8

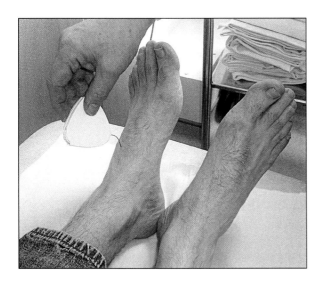

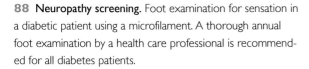

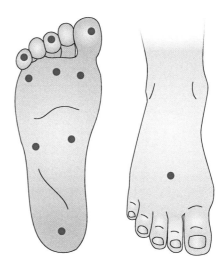

88 Neuropathy screening. Foot examination for sensation in a diabetic patient using a microfilament. A thorough annual foot examination by a health care professional is recommended for all diabetes patients.

89 Microfilament testing. The Semmes–Weinstein monofilament test is performed at 10 sites on the foot. The filament exerts 10 grams of force when bowed against the skin for one second. Patients who cannot reliably detect this are considered to have lost protective sensation.

Diabetic neuropathy

Chronic sensory polyneuropathy

◆ Diabetic neuropathies are usually sensory and most commonly bilateral, symmetrical, peripheral, and chronic (see **90**, next page).
  ◇ Chronic symmetrical sensory polyneuropathy is the most common form.
◆ Sensory deficits first appear in the distal lower extremities. A slowing in nerve conduction is the first physiological change, and occurs even before symptoms appear.
◆ Early clinical signs are impaired vibration sense (using a 128-Hz tuning fork), pain sensation (deep before superficial), paresthesias, and temperature sensation in the feet.
  ◇ At later stages patients may complain of a feeling of 'walking on cotton wool' and can lose their balance when washing the face or walking in the dark, owing to impaired proprioception.
◆ Involvement of the hands is much less common and results in a 'stocking and glove' sensory loss.
◆ Complications include unrecognized trauma at pressure points, beginning as blistering due to an ill-fitting shoe or a hot water bottle, and leading to ulceration.

◆ Unbalanced traction by the long flexor muscles leads to a characteristic foot, with a high arch and clawed toes.
  ◇ This change in turn leads to abnormal pressure distribution, resulting in callus formation under the first metatarsal head or on the tips of the toes and perforating neuropathic ulceration (see Chapter 8).
◆ Neuropathic arthropathy (Charcot's joints) may sometimes develop in any joint, but most often affects the ankle or mid-tarsal joints (see Chapter 8).

Early clinical signs of chronic sensory polyneuropathy are an impaired sense of vibration, pain, and temperature in the feet.

Clinical patterns of diabetic peripheral neuropathy

Syndrome	CHRONIC INSIDIOUS SENSORY NEUROPATHY	ACUTE PAINFUL NEUROPATHY
Pattern of presentation		
Sensory loss	+ → ++	+
Pain	0 → +++	+++
Tension reflexes	↓	↓
Muscle wasting and weakness	0 → ++	+ → +++
Autonomic features	+ → ++	May be present
Prevalence; relationship to glycemia; transience	Common; usually unrelated to glycemia	Relatively rare; onset often during hyperglycemia; transient

Acute sensory neuropathy

◆ Although some of the symptoms of acute and chronic sensory neuropathy are similar, there are differences in the mode of onset, signs, and prognosis (**90**). Acute neuropathies may be either:
  ◇ Diffuse and painful.
  ◇ Focal.
◆ In either event they are usually transient.
◆ A diffuse, painful neuropathy is uncommon (5%). The patient describes burning or crawling pains in the feet, shins and anterior thighs, muscular leg cramps, all typically worse at night, and pressure from bedclothes may be intolerable (allodynia). Painful neuropathy may present at diagnosis or develop after sudden improvement in glycemic control. It usually resolves spontaneously after 3 months and resolves in 90% of cases at 2 years.

◇ A more chronic form, developing later in the course of the disease, is sometimes resistant to almost all forms of therapy. There is no diagnostic test so alternative diagnoses such as vitamin B12 deficiency, alcohol, HIV-related, drug-related (isoniazid, nitrofurantoin), porphyria, and cancer-related neuropathy should be considered.
◇ Muscle wasting is not a feature and objective signs can be minimal.
◆ Focal mononeuritis and mononeuritis multiplex (multiple mononeuropathy) can affect any nerve in the body. Typically the onset is abrupt and sometimes painful.

Diabetic peripheral neuropathy can be acute or chronic.

PROXIMAL MOTOR MYOPATHY	DIFFUSE MOTOR NEUROPATHY	FOCAL NERVE PALSIES	
	Pressure	Not pressure	
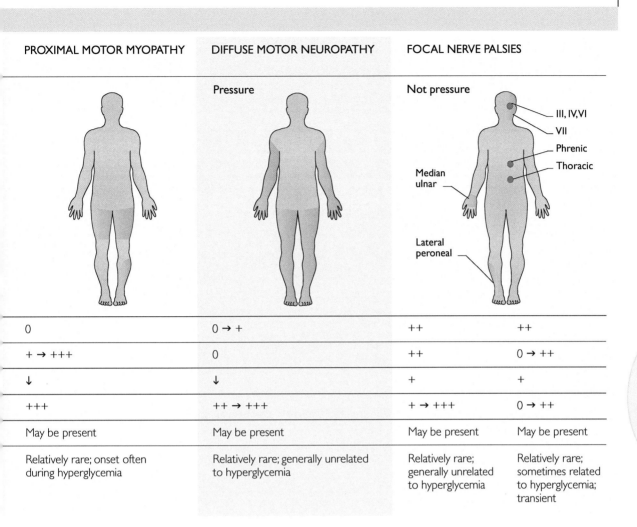			
0	0 → +	++	++
+ → +++	0	++	0 → ++
↓	↓	+	+
+++	++ → +++	+ → +++	0 → ++
May be present	May be present	May be present	May be present
Relatively rare; onset often during hyperglycemia	Relatively rare; generally unrelated to hyperglycemia	Relatively rare; generally unrelated to hyperglycemia	Relatively rare; sometimes related to hyperglycemia; transient

90 Clinical patterns. Note that different forms of diabetic neuropathy can coexist in the same patient.

◆ Isolated cranial nerve palsies are more commonly seen in the elderly and are rare in children.

◇ Involvement of the third cranial nerve is the most common, with characteristic pupillary sparing, i.e. pupillary reflexes are often retained owing to sparing of pupillomotor fibers. It usually presents with unilateral ophthalmoplegia that spares lateral eye movement, and pain above or behind the eye. However, pain may be absent or mild in half of the cases.

◇ The sixth cranial nerve is also commonly involved.

◇ The fourth and seventh cranial nerves are affected less often and not more frequently than in nondiabetic patients.

◇ Full spontaneous recovery is the rule for most episodes of focal cranial nerve involvement, even in the elderly.

◆ Isolated peripheral nerve palsies are more commonly seen in diabetic than nondiabetic individuals. Lesions are more likely to occur at sites for external pressure palsies or nerve entrapment (e.g. the median nerve in the carpal tunnel). Carpal tunnel syndrome is a common cause for sensory symptoms in the hands in diabetes, and is twice as common in diabetics than in nondiabetics.

◆ Radiculopathy (i.e. involvement of a spinal root) may occur. Thoracic radiculopathy presents as dermatomal pain and loss of sensation. Hypesthesia can occur. Spontaneous resolution usually occurs in 6–24 months.

Acute motor neuropathy

- Diabetic amyotrophy is a motor neuropathy which is rare and more prevalent in older men.
- It presents as weight loss, depression, and painful wasting of the quadriceps muscles.
    - ◇ Depression may be severe and resolves as the weight increases.
    - ◇ The wasting may be marked, causing severe proximal weakness, and knee reflexes may be diminished or absent. The affected area is often extremely tender.
    - ◇ Extensor plantar responses sometimes develop and cerebrospinal fluid (CSF) protein content is elevated.
    - ◇ The presentation may be unilateral; the contralateral thigh can be involved immediately following or months after the initial insult.
- Diabetic amyotrophy is usually associated with periods of poor glycemic control and may be present at diagnosis. It resolves like an acute sensory neuropathy with the same management regimen.
- Nondiabetic causes for the amyotrophy must be excluded, including spinal lesions.

Clinical manifestations of diabetic autonomic neuropathy

ORGAN SYSTEM	MANIFESTATION
Cardiovascular	Postural hypotension, tachycardia, sudden cardiac death
Gastrointestinal	Esophageal dysmotility, gastroparesis, diarrhea, constipation, incontinence
Genitourinary	Erectile dysfunction, retrograde ejaculation, bladder dysfunction
Neuroendocrine	Hypoglycemia unawareness
Sudomotor	Dry skin, impaired skin blood flow, gustatory sweating
Pupillary	Abnormal reflexes

91 Symptoms of autonomic neuropathy. Symptoms vary according to the nerves and organ systems affected.

Autonomic neuropathy

- Diabetic autonomic neuropathy (DAN) can affect almost every organ system (**91**). It affects both the sympathetic and parasympathetic nervous systems and can be disabling.
- Asymptomatic autonomic changes can be demonstrated on laboratory testing in many patients, but because of its variable manifestation, it can escape clinical recognition.
- Patients with severe autonomic neuropathy have an increased mortality possibly due to cardio-respiratory arrest, especially in those with marked prolongation of the QTc interval on ECG.

Cardiovascular system
- Autonomic neuropathy results in tachycardia at rest and loss of sinus arrhythmia. Cardiovascular reflexes including the Valsalva maneuver are impaired.
- A fixed heart rate that does not respond to exercise should alert one to cardiovascular autonomic neuropathy.
- Silent ischemia is more common in patients with DAN.
- Myocardial infarction should be entertained in diabetic patients with unexplained nausea, vomiting, or diaphoresis even if there is no chest pain.
- DAN is associated with impaired dilation of coronary arteries and can predispose to arrhythmias.
- Impaired blood pressure regulation is another manifestation of DAN.
    - ◇ The normal diurnal blood pressure variation is lost, so that patients have supine hypertension at night.
    - ◇ Postural hypotension, where there is an orthostatic fall in blood pressure by more than 30 mmHg, results from loss of sympathetic tone to peripheral and splanchnic arterioles. Patients complain of dizziness, feeling faint, blurring of vision, or loss of consciousness.

Diabetic autonomic neuropathy can escape clinical recognition because of its variable manifestation.

- Early cardiovascular DAN may not be clinically apparent, and may require diagnostic tests for evaluation. Most of these techniques rely on the impaired heart-rate variability and blood pressure responses.
  - ◇ The heart rate response to standing can be ascertained by continuous ECG monitoring. The R–R interval is then measured after standing at beats 15 and 30. The ratio of the R–R interval at beat 30:15 is normally >1.03 since a tachycardia is followed by reflex bradycardia.

Gastrointestinal tract

- Gastroparesis results in delayed gastric emptying. Solid-phase emptying occurs in the antrum, and if affected in diabetic patients, results in gastric retention.
  - ◇ Vagal neuropathy can cause gastroparesis, often asymptomatic, but sometimes resulting in intractable vomiting. Other milder symptoms are early satiety, nausea, bloatedness, and abdominal pain.
  - ◇ Scintigraphic gastric emptying studies are used to diagnose gastroparesis.
- Diarrhea often occurs at night with urgency and incontinence. Bacterial overgrowth in the stagnant bowel, pancreatic exocrine insufficiency, malabsorption, and incontinence can lead to diarrhea and steatorrhea.

Bladder involvement

- DAN can lead to decreased bladder sensation and reduced voiding frequency.
  - ◇ This can result in bladder enlargement, bladder stasis, loss of tone and incomplete emptying (predisposing to infection) with eventual urinary retention.
  - ◇ Patients experience dribbling and urinary incontinence.
  - ◇ A postvoiding residual of more than 150 ml indicates bladder dysfunction and can be ascertained by postvoiding catheterization or postvoiding ultrasonography.

Erectile dysfunction

- Erectile dysfunction is a common complication of diabetes resulting from autonomic neuropathy, vascular disease, or more often a combination of both. Acute illness, for whatever reason, can lead to transient impotence.
- A careful history should determine the nature of erectile dysfunction to establish the ability to obtain erections, penetration, and ejaculation, or combinations of these problems.
- Common presentations in diabetes are:
  - ◇ Incomplete erections.
  - ◇ Absent emissions due to retrograde ejaculation in patients with autonomic neuropathy.
- Erectile dysfunction in diabetes has many causes including anxiety, depression, alcohol excess, drugs, primary or secondary gonadal failure, and hypothyroidism, and is more common with age.
  - ◇ History and examination should focus on these possible causes.
  - ◇ Blood should be taken for luteinizing hormone (LH), follicle-stimulating hormone (FSH), testosterone, prolactin, and thyroid function.
- Sexual dysfunction is also a feature in women though the management has not yet been determined.

Neuroendocrine disturbances

- In patients with longstanding diabetes, there is loss of the adrenergic symptoms of hypoglycemia that usually precede neuroglycopenia. The counter-regulatory responses of glucagon and catecholamines are impaired.
- Patients have hypoglycemia unawareness, which increases the risk of going into a coma.

Sudomotor dysfunction

- Upper body hyperhidrosis and lower body anhidrosis are seen in DAN.
- Gustatory sweating (especially after cheese or wine) is an often unrecognized manifestation.
- The dry and cracked skin commonly seen in diabetes contributes to the development of skin infection.

Pupillary effects

- In DAN, there is decreased pupillary diameter in dark adaptation that might result in difficulty during night driving.

Diabetic neuropathy

Treatment and management

- The management of diabetic neuropathies depends on the nature of the neuropathy.

Acute sensory neuropathies

- The first step is to explore other nondiabetic causes.
- Once other conditions have been reasonably excluded, four factors are important:
  - ◇ Reassurance about the high likelihood of remission within months.
  - ◇ Management of blood glucose control, often with insulin even when glucose control is not bad.
  - ◇ Medications: the treatment of choice for acute painful neuropathy is pregabalin (recommended in the USA) or duloxetine (recommended in the UK), or, when such therapy is unsuccessful, both in combination. Other treatments include tricyclic antidepressants, gabapentin, and carbamazepine, which all reduce the perception of neuritic pain. Topical capsaicin-containing creams help some patients, but can discolor clothes. Epidurals may be required for chronic unremitting pain.
  - ◇ Many vitamins, including vitamin B, are used without clear evidence of their benefit.

Focal sensory mononeuropathies

- It is important first to explore nondiabetic causes.
- Once diabetes is identified as the likely cause, four factors are important:
  - ◇ Reassurance about the high likelihood of remission within months.
  - ◇ Management of blood glucose control, with the introduction of insulin should optimum control of either glucose or the pain be difficult.
  - ◇ Symptomatic relief such as eye patches for diplopia, or wrist splints for carpal tunnel syndrome.
  - ◇ Consider surgery for carpal tunnel syndrome and radiculopathy to decompress the lesions should pain not resolve.

Acute motor neuropathies

- Management is similar to that for acute mononeuropathies and includes:
  - ◇ Reassurance regarding likelihood of remission.
  - ◇ Blood glucose control using insulin therapy.
  - ◇ General care including bed rest when muscle wasting is severe.
  - ◇ Antidepressant therapy when the depression is severe.

Autonomic neuropathy

Cardiovascular system

- Patients with orthostatic hypotension should be instructed not to get up suddenly from a reclining position.
- The use of Jobst stockings in the waking hours helps to increase venous return from the periphery and alleviate orthostatic hypotension.
- Debilitating hypotension can be helped by ephedrine or midodrine, or fludrocortisone. Treatment has to be adjusted to minimize symptoms and at the same time avoid the development of supine hypertension or congestive heart failure.

Gastrointestinal tract

- Optimization of blood glucose levels can improve gastric motility.
- Frequent small meals with reduced fat content helps in gastroparesis.
- Metoclopramide and domperidone (not available in the US) have antiemetic effects and are helpful in gastroparesis. Erythromycin stimulates motilin receptors, and improves gastric emptying.
- Broad-spectrum antibiotics such as doxycycline or metronidazole are good treatments for bacterial overgrowth and can improve diarrhea. The antidiarrheal drug loperamide and diphenoxylate offer symptomatic relief.
- A laparoscopically implanted gastric pacemaker can improve gastric emptying.

Erectile dysfunction is a common complication of diabetes. Patients require counseling as well as treatment.

Bladder involvement

◆ Urinary retention can be improved by cholinergic agents such as bethanechol.

◆ Incomplete bladder emptying leading to distention will benefit from intermittent catheterization.

◆ Urinary tract infections should be treated aggressively with antibiotics.

Erectile dysfunction

◆ All patients require counseling irrespective of the cause of the erectile dysfunction. Therapy for erectile dysfunction includes:

◇ Phosphodiesterase type-5 (PDE5) inhibitors. A therapeutic trial of these agents including sildenafil citrate (Viagra) should be considered in most impotent diabetic patients who do not suffer from angina or previous myocardial infarction (concurrent use of nitrates is a contraindication). These drugs enhance the effects of nitric oxide on smooth muscle and increase penile blood flow. About 60% of patients benefit (**92**). Side-effects, including headaches and altered vision, are not uncommon. If a PDE5 inhibitor succeeds it is worth trying without it after a few months, since sometimes potency will continue unaided after confidence is restored. Psychological factors are important and long-acting agents such as tadalafil can be helpful, as they reduce the need to plan precise treatment periods.

◇ Prostaglandin E-1 preparations. These agents promote penile blood flow when applied topically to the urethra or as an intracavernosal injection. Alprostadil given after suitable training via a small pellet inserted into the urethra has a lower success rate than intracavernosal injection of the same drug, but is less invasive. If the partner is pregnant, barrier contraception must be used to keep prostaglandin away from the fetus.

◇ Intracavernous injection. Patients can be trained to inject either alprostadil or papaverine (a smooth muscle relaxant), sometimes given with phentolamine and thymoxamine (alpha-adrenoreceptor blockers). The dose should be increased incrementally until a satisfactory response is obtained. Side-effects include local reactions (e.g. discomfort, hematoma, fibrosis) and priapism. Patients should be given contact details for urgent treatment should erection last for more than 3 hours. To treat priapism, insert a large butterfly needle into the cavernous tissue and aspirate blood with a large syringe until detumescence has occurred.

◇ Vacuum devices. These provide a non-pharmacological aid. A perspex tube with a seal in the base is placed over the penis and a vacuum pump draws blood into the penis to achieve tumescence, which is then maintained by slipping a rubber band over the base of the penis (then removing the tube) until intercourse is complete.

Diabetic neuropathy

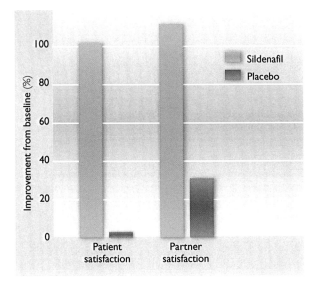

92 Oral therapy for erectile dysfunction. Sildenafil (Viagra) is usually regarded as a first-line drug for the treatment of erectile dysfunction. Response rates against placebo are high, with over 60% success in trials.

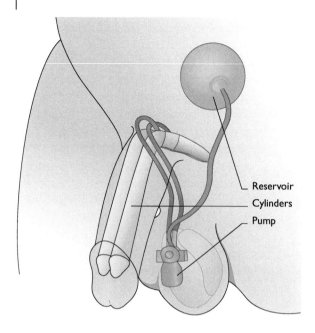

93 Penile implant surgery. There are a number of prosthetic options available: this shows a three-piece inflatable implant consisting of a pair of cylinders implanted in the penis, a pump bulb implanted in the scrotum, and a reservoir placed within the abdomen.

Reservoir
Cylinders
Pump

◇ Surgery. A proportion of patients find none of these solutions of value, especially if they have vascular disease. Patients with erectile dysfunction unresponsive to drug therapy can achieve penetration by means of a semirigid plastic rod inserted surgically into the penis. Other more sophisticated devices can generate an erect penis when required, using a hydraulic system (**93**).

◇ Constriction of venous outflow. Constriction of venous outflow from the penis by application of an elastic band around the base of the penis can enhance the firmness of an erection, but on its own will lead to an engorged penis without unidirectional rigidity (the so-called 'wand' effect). Whether application of a constricting band in association with a PDE5 inhibitor will enhance the success of the latter remains to be proven, but it may be worthwhile as a trial.

CHAPTER 8

The diabetic foot

Overview

◆ Diabetic foot problems are responsible for nearly 50% of all diabetes-related hospital bed-days.

◆ Ten to fifteen percent of diabetic patients develop foot ulcers at some stage in their lives.

◆ Fifty percent of all lower limb amputations are performed on people with diabetes.

◆ The risk of amputation is increased 15-fold in diabetes. That risk has declined substantially in the last 30 years but is still particularly high in those on dialysis (about 60 per 1000 person-years) or those with a history of foot ulceration (about 15 per 1000 person-years).

◆ Conservative management of foot problems has dramatically reduced the risk of amputation by simple procedures such as good footwear, chiropody, cleanliness, aggressive surgical debridement, and ulcer management. Even that most dramatic of diabetic foot problems, Charcot's arthropathy (see p. 103), no longer means an inevitable progression to amputation.

◆ Diabetic foot problems are not only an important complication, but they are also a preventable complication.

Pathophysiology and risk factors

◆ The impact of diabetes complications mediated through micro- and macrovascular disease is nowhere better exemplified than by the feet:

◇ All the risk factors, especially hyperglycemia, that are important to microvascular disease predispose to peripheral neuropathy and increase the risk of foot problems by disturbing the foot structure, physiology, and immune responses to trauma and infection.

◇ Those same risk factors, but especially dyslipidemia, smoking, and hypertension, that predispose to macrovascular disease also increase the risk of foot problems by disturbing the foot physiology, blood supply, and immune responses to trauma and infection.

◆ The major underlying causes of diabetic foot disease are:

◇ Peripheral neuropathy.
◇ Peripheral arterial disease.
◇ Infection secondary to trauma or ulceration.
◇ High plantar pressure.
◇ Deformities.

Neuropathy

◆ *Motor neuropathy.* Loss of neural supply to the intrinsic muscles of the foot leads to an imbalance between the flexor and extensor mechanisms, clawing of the toes, and increased prominence of the metatarsal heads.

◆ *Autonomic neuropathy.* Loss of sweat gland function leads to dry skin predisposed to skin cracking and infection. Loss of peripheral sympathetic vascular tone increases distal arterial flow and may lead to edema and osteopenia.

◆ *Sensory neuropathy.* Diminished sensibility to pain means that poorly-fitting shoes or early signs of foot deformity or lesions may go unnoticed by the patient and uncorrected. Callus is prevalent in neuropathic ulcers and reduces the healing potential of an ulcer, predisposing to infection.

Diabetic foot problems are preventable.

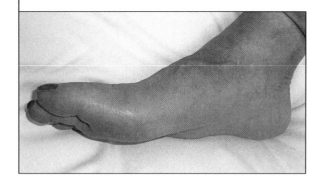

94 Neuropathic foot. Disrupted foot structure associated with Charcot's arthropathy. Note the distended veins associated with arteriovenous shunt.

Peripheral arterial disease

◆ Reduced blood supply mimics and exacerbates the changes brought about by neuropathy.

◆ Occlusive arterial disease also results in hypoxia and reduced wound healing with increased infection risk.

◆ Persistent hyperglycemia results in endothelial cell dysfunction and smooth cell abnormalities in peripheral arteries.

◆ In Charcot's arthropathy there is an arteriovenous shunt across the foot with distended dorsal veins (Ward's sign) (**94**).

Infection

◆ The damage resulting from neuropathy, ischemia, trauma, or all three predisposes to infection. Infection may be bacterial (in association with ulcers) or fungal (especially of toe nails).

Pressure

◆ Repetitive pressure, shear from walking and weight bearing, or inappropriate footwear, leads to increased plantar pressures, inducing callus formation and skin breakdown.

Clinical presentation and evaluation

◆ Systematic examination, evaluation, and appropriate categorization of foot ulcers will provide a guide to treatment and prognosis (**95**, **96**, **97**).

Evaluation

◆ All patients with diabetes should receive a thorough foot examination at least once a year; those with diabetic foot-related complaints should be evaluated more frequently. Patients are often unaware of serious foot problems because of the masking effect of neuropathy.

Clinical features of neuropathic vs ischemic foot ulcer

NEUROPATHIC ULCER	ISCHEMIC ULCER
Sensory defect	Not necessarily a sensory defect
Pulses present	Pulses absent
Subluxed metatarsal heads (cocked toes)	Foot structure retained
Ulceration of pressure points	Ulceration at points of ischemia, not pressure
Punched-out deep ulcer with surrounding callus	Superficial ulcers without callus

Wagner ulcer classification

GRADE	CLINICAL PRESENTATION
0	No open lesions; may have deformity or cellulitis
1	Superficial ulcer
2	Ulcer extension involving ligaments, tendon, joint capsule or fascia without abscess or osteomyelitis
3	Deep ulcer or osteomyelitis
4	Gangrene to portion of forefoot
5	Extensive gangrene of foot

95 Evaluating an ulcer in the diabetic foot. Ischemia and neuropathy can be difficult to differentiate; a thorough assessment is important.

96 Ulcer classification. Systematic evaluation and categorization of foot ulcers help guide appropriate treatment. The Wagner system is the most commonly used.

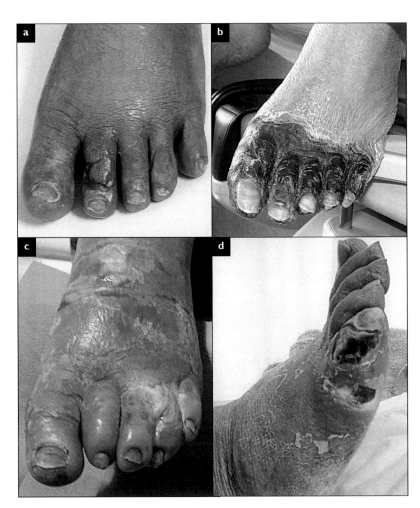

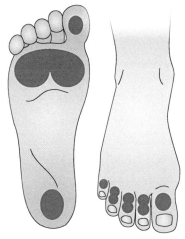

97 Diabetic foot ulcers. (a) Ischemic ulcer: digital ischemia is seen in the second toe. (b) Extensive ischemia affects all toes back to the level of the midfoot. (c) A neuropathic lesion at the base of the fourth toe has been the point of entry of extensive cellulitis of the whole foot. (d) Mixed neuro–ischemic lesion affecting the small toe. Below: neuropathic lesions tend to occur on plantar surfaces and ischemic ones over bone prominences.

The diabetic foot

Examination

◆ The following should be inspected/examined:
  ◇ *Footwear:* type; fit; pattern; foreign bodies.
  ◇ *Foot:* structure; distortion, e.g. Charcot's; pressure points; infection or ulcers between the toes; nails (for infection, length and whether ingrowing).
  ◇ *Skin:* whether dry; presence of fissures or calluses.
  ◇ *Vessels:* pulses; venous filling time; color.
  ◇ *Nerves:* examine sensors (reflexes, vibration, temperature, pain); motors (muscle power, muscle atrophy).
◆ Referral to a podiatrist (chiropodist) or foot clinic is recommended when patients manifest certain foot changes (**98**).
  ◇ In some services, patients with established neuropathy are offered regular monitoring by podiatry; this may be especially important for patients with visual impairment.

Indications for referral

Callus, corns or ingrowing toenails

Ulcer

Significant ischemia

Anatomical abnormality

Amputation or previous ulcer

Charcot's arthropathy

98 Referral criteria. These six features identified by a clinician should prompt referral to an appropriate specialist, e.g. podiatrist (callus, anatomical abnormality) or podiatrist plus specialist foot clinic for all other conditions.

Principles of foot care

Footwear must be carefully measured and checked regularly for foreign objects
Shoes should preferably be lace-up shoes or trainers
Feet should be washed daily and dried well especially between the toes
Toenails should be cut straight across, carefully and regularly
Feet should be inspected daily especially on the soles
Moisturizing creams are to be used for calluses or fissures
Refer to podiatrist when appropriate

99 Foot care. Simple management procedures for foot problems dramatically reduce the risk of amputation.

Treatment and management

◆ Since diabetic foot problems are, by and large, preventable, it is important to learn the principles of foot care (**99**).

◆ Several conditions put the foot at risk of amputations, and should be addressed to prevent progression.

◇ The five main threats to skin and subcutaneous tissues in the foot are neuropathy, peripheral arterial disease, infection, high plantar pressure, and deformities. Ulcer management centers on these five aspects of care and will typically involve several disciplines including a physician, a podiatrist, and a surgeon (usually vascular or orthopedic) (**100**).

100 Risk levels. The risk of diabetic foot can be stratified and resources prioritized according to need. *Adapted from the SCI-DC foot risk stratification tool.*

Assess foot pulses, monofilament sensation, history of foot ulcer, presence of foot deformity, and ability to self-care

LOW RISK

No risk factors
• No sensation loss: able to feel 10g monofilament
• No signs of peripheral vascular disease
• No foot deformity or previous ulcer

MODERATE RISK

One risk factor
• Loss of sensation: unable to feel monofilament
OR
• Signs of peripheral vascular disease: unable to detect pulses in a foot
OR
• Callus/deformity
OR
• Unable to see/reach foot

HIGH RISK

• Previous ulceration or amputation
OR
More than one risk factor
• Loss of sensation: unable to feel monofilament
AND
• Signs of peripheral vascular disease: absent pulses
OR
• One of above with callus/deformity

ACTIVE DISEASE

Presence of:
• Active ulceration
• Spreading infection
• Critical ischemia
• Gangrene
• Unexplained swelling and inflammation, with or without pain

Action
• Annual screening by healthcare professional
• Self-management
• Patient education
• Emergency contact numbers

Action
• Annual screening by healthcare professional
• Self-management
• Patient education
• Emergency contact numbers

Action
• Annual screening by healthcare professional
• Self-management
• Patient education
• Emergency contact numbers

Action
• Rapid referral to and management by a member of multidisciplinary team
• Self-management
• Patient education
• Emergency contact numbers
• Referral for specialist intervention when required

Infection

◆ Infections in diabetes should be managed intensively by identifying the relevant organism and using early and aggressive antibiotic treatment.
  ◇ *Streptococcus pyogenes, Staphylococcus aureus*, and anaerobic species are prevalent.
◆ Since infections may lead to loss of glycemic control, and are a common cause of ketoacidosis, insulin-treated patients need to increase their dose in the face of infection, and noninsulin-treated patients may need insulin therapy when they have an infection.
◆ Therapy includes ulcer debridement, callus removal, protection of pressure points, and antibiotics.
  ◇ Antibiotics must be broad spectrum, moderately high dosage, given for prolonged periods often in excess of 1 month until infection is resolved.
◆ For deep or chronic infections, radiography of the feet may be required to exclude osteomyelitis (**101**). If doubt remains about osteomyelitis, a magnetic resonance imaging (MRI), computed tomography (CT), or gallium bone scan may provide further evidence.
  ◇ Sequential radiography (e.g. at intervals of 2 weeks apart) may be needed to clarify the situation.
  ◇ Radiological diagnosis of osteomyelitis can be complex given that in an infected diabetic foot there may be areas of demineralization in bones that are not directly infected, and this topic is beyond the scope of this book.
  ◇ Although the gold standard for diagnosis of osteomyelitis is bone biopsy, this is rarely used due to the hazards of the procedure.
◆ Osteomyelitis can be treated with long-term intravenous antibiotics – at least 6 weeks – but may require excision of the infected bone. Arterial revascularization may assist healing.
◆ In patients who decline amputation, antibiotics may contain even osteomyelitis for several months (or even years). However, this is not recommended since chronic infection promotes a systemic catabolic and proinflammatory state that affects the patient's well-being.

Peripheral arterial disease

◆ The blood flow to the feet is assessed clinically, with Doppler ultrasound, or when severe and surgery is contemplated, by femoral arteriography.
  ◇ Arterial calcification will give false Doppler readings suggesting high blood flow.
  ◇ Localized areas of occlusion as shown on arteriography may be amenable to bypass surgery, stents, or angioplasty, or *in extremis* to amputation.

Ulcer management typically involves several disciplines.

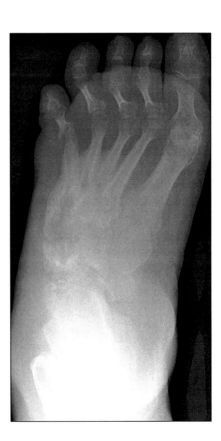

101 Osteomyelitis. Radiograph of a left foot, showing bone destruction and periosteal bone formation, most notably in the 5th metatarsal. *Courtesy Barts and The London Hospital Trust.*

The diabetic foot

High plantar pressure

- Appropriate foot care, removal of callus formation, rest, and, when ulcerated, keeping the ulcerated site nonweight bearing, are essential.
  - ◇ A moisturizing cream can be used prophylactically to callus.
- Deep shoes and specially constructed insoles help to move pressure away from critical sites, while lightweight supports (e.g. 'air-boots' or 'foot casts') limit pressure on the feet.
- Recommence weight bearing gradually, preferably with specially crafted footwear, or, as a less satisfactory alternative, with sports trainers.

Deformities

- Deformities can be managed by appropriate foot wear or, if required, surgery.

The wound environment

- Dressings are used both to absorb exudate and to maintain moisture; in addition, they protect the wound from contamination.
- New techniques to promote healing of chronic ulceration are available but there is a paucity of evidence relating to their effectiveness. They are expensive (e.g. hyperbaric oxygen or growth factors) and their role is yet to be established.
  - ◇ Hydrogel dressings, hyberbaric oxygen therapy, and larval therapy have some evidence for efficacy.
  - ◇ There is perhaps less evidence for alginate-based dressings, platelet-derived growth factors, negative pressure wound therapy, dimethyl sulfoxide dressings, and cultured dermis; the latter is like a skin graft but constructed from neonatal fibroblasts embedded in a synthetic matrix.

Surgery

- Amputations need to be undertaken at the appropriate time. They are the definitive treatment of osteomyelitis, but a trial of antibiotics (with or without soft-tissue debridement) will usually precede amputation.
  - ◇ Amputation should be avoided, where possible, as it has long-term implications for the patient, both physiological and psychological.
- Amputations can be:
  - ◇ Local, involving a ray excision of the second, third or fourth toe and the associated metatarsal.
  - ◇ More radical, including above- or below-knee amputations of the limb.
- Sometimes an angioplasty will be required to improve blood supply before amputation is attempted.
  - ◇ When multiple levels of occlusion are present, revascularization at each point is necessary to restore arterial blood flow.
  - ◇ Transluminal angioplasty of the iliac arteries allied to surgical bypass in the distal extremity may be valuable.
- Amputation inevitably changes the biomechanics of the limb(s) that remain and will necessitate a review of footwear after recovery from the procedure.
  - ◇ The effort required to walk with a prosthesis is high and may be too much for the elderly, who are then confined to a wheelchair.
  - ◇ The shift in weight can promote ulceration in the contralateral limb.

The key components of ulcer management include avoiding pressure, treating infection, improving circulation, and promoting healing.

Amputation has long-term implications and should be avoided if possible.

Charcot's arthropathy

◆ Charcot's arthropathy results from a dense peripheral sensory neuropathy. It was originally described as a feature of syphilis and leprosy, but the most common cause today is diabetes. The structure of the foot (though any large joint can be affected) is lost, accompanied by bone thinning and small fractures. Subsequently, the joints of the feet are disrupted and disorganized and the abnormal structure is subject to further distortion, pressure points, ulceration, and joint instability (**102**, **103**, **104**).

◆ There are two main classifications of Charcot neuroarthropathy (Eichenholz and Brodsky), which describe disease progress and distribution, respectively.

◆ The Eichenholz classification describes the evolution of the condition over time:
  ◇ Stage 1: destruction.
  ◇ Stage 2: coalescence.
  ◇ Stage 3: consolidation.

◆ A 'stage 0' has also come into use to classify the swollen, hot, usually rather painful foot in which plain foot radiograph is normal but MRI shows bone edema and stress fractures.

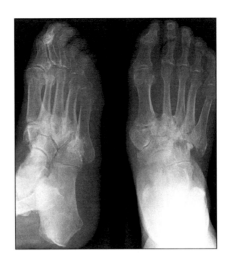

102 **Charcot's arthropathy.** Radiograph showing destruction and coalescence of the tarsometatarsal region (where the process usually starts) of the right foot. *Photo courtesy Barts and The London Hospital Trust..*

◆ Management of Charcot's arthropathy includes:
  ◇ Immobilization.
  ◇ Custom-made footwear.
  ◇ Reconstruction (including realignment of unstable joints).
  ◇ Intravenous bisphosphonates (which suppress osteoclast activity).
◆ The key to management is early diagnosis and reduction of pressure.

The diabetic foot

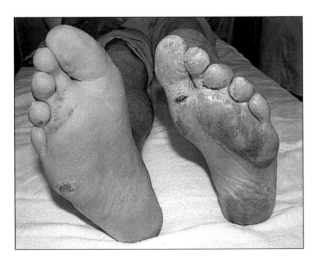

103 **Charcot's arthropathy.** A patient with neuropathic feet bilaterally; the right foot showing changes of Charcot's arthropathy along its lateral border, with an overlying ulcer. The left foot shows callus formation.

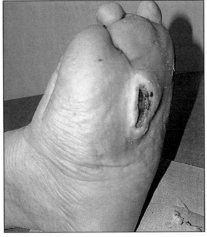

104 **Charcot's arthropathy.** An 'end-stage' Charcot's foot with previous amputations and a severely distorted foot structure with marked callus around a neuropathetic ulcer.

CHAPTER 9

Diabetic eye disease

Overview

◆ Patients with diabetes are at risk of eye disease including:
  ◇ **Retinopathy**. About 5% of patients in the past became blind after 30 years of diabetes, and diabetes is the commonest cause of blindness in the population up to 65 years of age.
  ◇ **Maculopathy**. Increased permeability of the capillaries and microaneurysms in the retina can result in accumulation of fluid and thickening in the macular area.
  ◇ **Cataracts**. The lens may be affected by reversible osmotic changes in patients with acute hyperglycemia, causing blurred vision. Senile cataracts develop 10 years earlier in diabetic patients, compared to nondiabetic subjects.
  ◇ **Glaucoma**. Glaucoma is more prevalent in diabetes due to new vessel formation in the iris (rubeosis iridis). Open-angle glaucoma is not more prevalent in diabetes.
  ◇ **Ocular nerve palsies**. Ocular palsies of the third and sixth cranial nerves can occur. Like other causes of mononeuritis, these palsies are acute and transient, always resolving within 2 years and usually within 4 months.

Natural history

◆ Duration of diabetes is one of the best predictors of retinopathy:
  ◇ Patients who have had type 1 diabetes for 5 years or less rarely have evidence of retinopathy.
  ◇ After 5–10 years of diabetes, close to 30% of type 1 diabetes patients have retinopathy.
  ◇ After 20–30 years, about 95% of patients have retinopathy, and 30–60% of these progress to sight-threatening proliferative retinopathy (**105**).
◆ In type 2 diabetes, 20% of newly diagnosed patients already have diabetic retinopathy, and most will subsequently develop the condition.
◆ Without treatment, 50% of patients with proliferative retinopathy become blind within 5 years.

Retinopathy is more likely with increasing duration of diabetes.

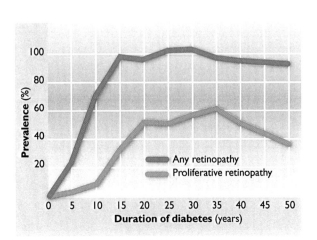

105 Prevalence of diabetic retinopathy in type 1 diabetes. Data from the Wisconsin Epidemiologic Study of Diabetic Retinopathy (WESDR) reported by Klein *et al.* showed that by 25 years following the onset of the disease, almost all patients had developed some sort of retinopathy, with over 50 percent having vision-threatening proliferative retinopathy.

Recommended ophthalmologic examination

TYPE I DIABETES

First examination within 3–5 years after diagnosis of diabetes once patient is age 10 years or older (since some evidence suggests that prepubertal duration of diabetes may be important in the development of microvascular complications, use clinical judgment)

Yearly routine follow-up at the minimum (more frequent if abnormal findings)

TYPE 2 DIABETES

First examination at the time of diagnosis of diabetes

Yearly routine follow-up at the minimum (more frequent if abnormal findings)

PREGNANCY IN PRE-EXISTING DIABETES

First examination prior to conception, then during first trimester

Follow-up is at physician discretion pending results of first-trimester examination

RETINOPATHY AND MACULAR EDEMA

Ophthalmology referral in patients with macular edema, severe NPDR, or any form of PDR

106 Eye examinations. Regular screening is important in order to detect early changes indicative of retinopathy.

107 Classification. Diabetic retinopathy is classed according to increasing severity. Recognition of the major subdivisions is important in terms of appropriate management, though these vary according to different classifications.

◆ Regular dilated eye examinations are recommended (**106**).
◆ Diabetic retinopathy can be classified into nonproliferative (NPDR) and proliferative (PDR).
  ◇ NPDR comprises: microaneurysms, 'dot and blot' hemorrhages, hard exudates, 'cotton-wool spots', intraretinal microvascular abnormalities (IRMAs), while venous beading, neovascularization, vitreous/preretinal hemorrhages, and traction-induced retinal detachment can be found in PDR (**107**).

Nonproliferative diabetic retinopathy

◆ Diabetic retinopathy is caused by progressive damage to the blood vessels that supply the retinal tissues (**108, 109**). Early changes are detectable by fluorescein angiography (**110**).
  ◇ Hyperglycemia leads to tissue hypoxia and reduced retinal function.
  ◇ Leucocyte adhesion to the capillary wall results in occlusion and reduced blood flow, and ultimately greater hypoxia and ischemia.
  ◇ Capillary nonperfusion can also cause compensatory dilation and microaneurysms in other vessels.
  ◇ Basement membrane thickening, endothelial cell damage, and degeneration of the pericytes supporting the blood vessel wall, cause breakdown of the blood–retina barrier and increased permeability of the retinal capillaries.
  ◇ Leakage of plasma, proteins, and growth factors such as VEGF, gives rise to cell edema and new vessel growth, respectively.

Classification of diabetic retinopathy

NONPROLIFERATIVE (NPDR)

Mild	• At least 1 microaneurysm
Moderate	• Hemorrhages or microaneurysms (H/Ma) • Soft exudates, venous beading (VB) and IRMAs definitely present
Severe	• H/Ma in all 4 quadrants • VB in 2 or more quadrants • IRMA in at least 1 quadrant

PROLIFERATIVE (PDR)

Low-risk	• New vessels on the retina
High-risk	• New vessels on the disc (NVD) of >25% of the disc area *OR* • Any NVD and vitreous or preretinal hemorrhage

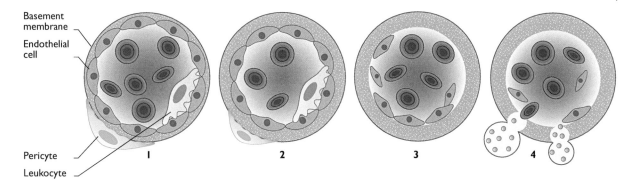

Basement membrane
Endothelial cell
Pericyte
Leukocyte

1   2   3   4

108 Capillary changes. (1) Leukocyte adhesion; (2) basement membrane thickening and reduced blood flow; (3) pericyte and endothelial cell death; (4) increased permeability.

◆ In NPDR, hemorrhages and microaneurysms can be seen:
  ◇ Clinically, microaneurysms are visible through the ophthalmoscope as round dots.
  ◇ By 20 years of diabetes, virtually all fundi show at least the occasional microaneurysm on ophthalmoscopy.
  ◇ When a microaneurysm ruptures, it may give rise to flame-shaped hemorrhages if in the superficial layers of the retina, or to 'dot and blot' hemorrhages in the deeper layers. The 'dot and blot' hemorrhages might be difficult to distinguish from microaneurysms just by using the ophthalmoscope.
◆ Exudation of fluid rich in lipids and protein causes hard exudates to form. These have a bright yellow–white color with an irregular outline and a sharply defined margin.
◆ In more advanced stages of NPDR, cotton-wool spots, venous beading and loops, and IRMAs can be seen. These features are associated with a high risk of progression to PDR and are sometimes termed 'preproliferative retinopathy'.
  ◇ Cotton-wool spots appear as gray or white fluffy-looking lesions in the nerve fiber layer of the retina that result from nerve fiber infarction, and are also a feature of hypertensive retinopathy.
  ◇ Venous beading denotes sluggish circulation in the retina.
  ◇ IRMAs are dilated capillaries shunting blood through nonperfused areas.

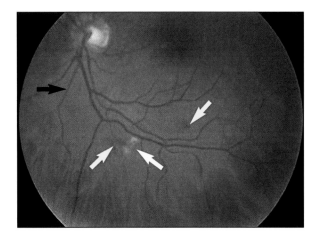

109 Moderate nonproliferative diabetic retinopathy. Retinal fundus photograph showing IRMA (black arrow), hemorrhages (yellow arrows), and cotton-wool spots (white arrow).

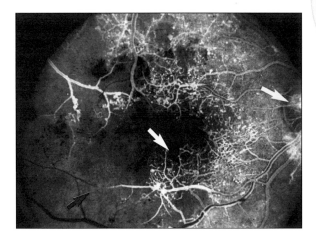

110 Fluorescein angiography. This photograph shows retinal ischemia and capillary nonperfusion (red arrow), micro-aneurysms, and vascular pruning (white arrow). There is an area of neovascularization on the optic nerve (yellow arrow), which is often associated with extensive retinal ischemia.
Courtesy Michael J. Tolentino, Center of Retina and Macular Disease, Winter Haven, Florida.

Diabetic eye disease

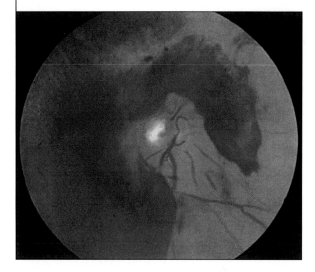

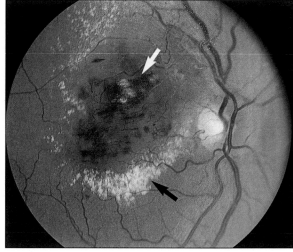

111 **Vitreous hemorrhage.** If vitreous hemorrhage is associated with visible neovascularization, this is considered high-risk PDR and would require panretinal photocoagulation. *Courtesy Rishi P. Singh, Cole Eye Institute, Cleveland Clinic.*

112 **Maculopathy.** Retinal fundus photograph showing exudates (black arrow), hemorrhage (yellow arrow), and edema in the area of the macula. *Courtesy Rishi P. Singh, Cole Eye Institute, Cleveland Clinic.*

Proliferative diabetic retinopathy

◆ In PDR, new blood vessels grow on the retinal surface in response to growth factors released from ischemic areas. These new vessels are fragile and bleed easily, so PDR is characterized by neovascularization, vitreous hemorrhage (**111**), or retinal detachment.
  ◇ The neovascularization often arises from retinal veins, and may be seen on or near the optic disc (NVD) or elsewhere (NVE). New vessels either are superficial on the retina or grow forward into the vitreous.
  ◇ Hemorrhages can be preretinal or vitreous. A vitreous hemorrhage can cause loss of vision. Ophthalmoscopy shows a featureless, gray haze. Partial recovery of vision is the rule as the blood is reabsorbed, but repeat bleeding may occur.
  ◇ Fibrous proliferation associated with new vessel formation can distort the retina and the vision. Such changes may give rise to traction bands that contract, producing retinal detachment.

Diabetic maculopathy

◆ Maculopathy is retinal damage concentrated at the macula, which can threaten central vision. It is a particular characteristic of type 2 diabetes.
◆ There are three types of maculopathy:
  ◇ Exudative.
  ◇ Edematous.
  ◇ Ischemic.
◆ Of these types, edematous may be difficult to visualize with direct ophthalmoscopy and ischemic is the least responsive to laser therapy.
◆ Macular edema (**112**) is the first feature of maculopathy and may in itself cause permanent macular damage, if not treated early. It can result in deterioration of visual acuity – especially if the fovea centralis is involved – even in the absence of significant findings by ophthalmoscopy, since retinal thickening is not easily detected by this method.
  ◇ Diabetic macular edema can be seen in any level of diabetic retinopathy.
◆ It is essential to screen diabetes patients regularly for changes in visual acuity.

Cataracts

◆ Cataract is characterized by a gradual clouding of the lens; senile cataracts are the most common form. Cataracts are 60% more common in diabetic than in nondiabetic patients.

◆ Cataracts result in reduced visual acuity that cannot be improved by viewing through a pin-hole. In the early stages they are usually asymptomatic, but if left untreated can cause blindness.

◆ Myotonic dystrophy and steroid therapy, which are associated with increased risk of diabetes, are in turn associated with cataracts.

◆ Juvenile or 'snowflake' cataracts are rare (about 1%), diffuse, rapidly progressive cataracts associated with very poorly controlled diabetes and amenable to surgery.

◆ Posterior subcapsular cataracts are more common in diabetic than nondiabetic patients.

◆ It is thought that with hyperglycemia, glucose in the aqueous humor enters the lens cells, is converted to sorbitol, and leads to osmotic swelling.

Glaucoma

◆ Neovascularization of the iris that can lead to neovascular glaucoma is a potentially serious ophthalmological complication in diabetes. New iris vessels form at the pupillary border, then progress into the angle of the anterior chamber.

◆ Neovascular glaucoma occurs when there is closure of the angle by the fibrovascular structures.

◆ Diabetes is the second leading cause of neo-vascular glaucoma.

Ocular nerve palsies

◆ Third nerve palsies are the most common cranial neuropathy in diabetes. Pupillary sparing is characteristic in diabetes, with preservation of the pupillary reflexes.

◆ External ocular palsies of the sixth nerve can also occur.

◆ Like other causes of mononeuritis, these palsies are acute and transient, almost always resolving within 2 years and usually within 4 months.
  ◇ Some 10% are bilateral or multiple and they can recur.

Treatment and management

◆ Medical treatment to limit diabetic eye disease development or progression involves aggressive treatment of blood glucose and blood pressure levels.

◆ In the DCCT, type 1 diabetic patients who were in the intensive glycemic control group had a 76% reduction in the rate of development of any retinopathy in those who did not have retinopathy at baseline (primary prevention cohort) and a 54% reduction in progression in those with established retinopathy (secondary intervention cohort) compared with the conventional treatment group.

◆ The benefit of tight glycemic control has been demonstrated for type 2 diabetes as well.
  ◇ In the UKPDS, there was a 21% reduction in the 1-year rate of progression of retinopathy.

◆ There is currently no specific medical treatment for diabetic retinopathy.
  ◇ Based on the Early Treatment Diabetic Retinopathy Study (ETDRS), aspirin treatment does not alter the progression of retinopathy.
  ◇ Smoking worsens the rate of retinopathy progression.
  ◇ Some evidence suggests that ACEIs are of particular value in hypertension and the threshold for introduction of these agents should be low.
  ◇ Intravitreal anti-vascular endothelial growth factor (anti-VEGF) injections have proved valuable in clinically significant macular edema.

◆ Development or progression of retinopathy may be accelerated by a sudden, rapid improvement in glycemic control, pregnancy, and in those with nephropathy; these groups need frequent monitoring.

Diabetic eye disease

Sudden improvement in glucose levels can accelerate retinopathy.

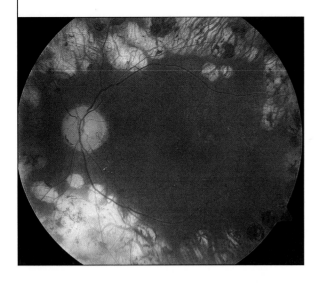

113 Laser treatment. Retinal fundus photograph of laser photocoagulation for proliferative diabetic retinopathy. *Courtesy Rishi P. Singh, Cole Eye Institute, Cleveland Clinic.*

◆ All patients with retinopathy should be examined regularly by a diabetologist or ophthalmologist. The ophthalmologist may perform fluorescein angiography to define the extent of the problem.
◆ Early referral is essential in the following circumstances:
   ◇ Deteriorating visual acuity.
   ◇ Hard exudates encroaching on the macula.
   ◇ Preproliferative changes (cotton-wool spots or venous beading).
   ◇ New vessel formation.
   ◇ Acute vitreous hemorrhage.
◆ Maculopathy and proliferative retinopathy are often treatable by retinal laser photocoagulation (**113**); in the latter condition, early effective therapy reduces the risk of visual loss by about 50%. Treatment of NVD is particularly successful using panretinal photocoagulation.
◆ Surgery can be performed to try to salvage vision after vitreous hemorrhage and to treat traction-induced retinal detachment.
◆ Visual aids should be considered for all patients with reduced vision. These include insulin injection pens, talking glucose meters, powerful illumination, magnifying glasses, audiobooks, and guide dogs. Support systems for the visually impaired can be contacted, including charitable organizations and occupational therapy centers.

Diabetic maculopathy
◆ Patients should be referred to a specialist if there is an unexplained change in visual acuity or hard exudates within two disc diameters of visual fixation.
◆ Patients with clinically significant macular edema may benefit from focal laser photocoagulation.
◆ The use of the anti-VEGF agents pegaptanib (Macugen) or bevacizumab (Avastin) is promising, especially for people who present late or in whom laser treatment has failed.

Cataracts
◆ In the UKPDS, intensive glycemic control was associated with a 34% reduction in cataract extraction compared to conventional treatment.
◆ The patient should be referred to a specialist for cataract removal when loss of vision interferes with their daily life.
◆ Cataract surgery with intraocular lens implantation is successful 90–95% of the time in restoring vision.
◆ Patients should be carefully selected since there are potential complications in diabetic patients.
   ◇ After cataract surgery in diabetic patients, there is an increased incidence of neovascularization of the iris and of neovascular glaucoma.
   ◇ In the presence of active proliferative retinopathy, care must be exercised given the risk of deterioration of the retinopathy. In this instance, laser therapy may have to be given concurrently.

Glaucoma
◆ The treatment of neovascularization of the iris and neovascular glaucoma may include a combination of the following: photocoagulation, topical and systemic antiglaucoma drugs, topical steroids, topical atropine, filtration surgery.

All patients with retinopathy should have a regular ophthalmic examination.

CHAPTER 10

Diabetic kidney disease

Overview

- The kidney can be damaged by diabetes in three main ways:
  - ◇ Glomerular damage.
  - ◇ Ischemia resulting from hypertrophy of afferent and efferent arterioles.
  - ◇ Ascending infection.
- Clinically significant nephropathy usually appears between 15 and 25 years after diagnosis and rarely develops >30 years from diagnosis.
- Nephropathy affects 25–35% of patients diagnosed under the age of 30, but recent data suggests this percentage is falling. It is the main cause of renal failure in Europe, accounting for more than 30% (40% in the US) of new renal replacement therapy.
  - ◇ Some ethnic groups, such as Native Americans, African-Americans, and South Asians are at particular risk.
- Patients with type 2 diabetes develop nephropathy less frequently than those with type 1 diabetes, however more than 80% of patients who do need renal replacement in the US have type 2 diabetes, since this is much more prevalent than type 1.
- Both proteinuria and diabetic nephropathy are associated with an increased risk of developing macrovascular disease.
- There is a strong genetic effect predisposing to nephropathy.

Proteinuria is a marker of cardiovascular risk.

Glomerular capillary
- Urine
- Protein
- Red blood cell
- Epithelial cell
- Glomerular basement membrane
- Endothelial cell

114 Proteinuria. Thickening of the basement membrane is the earliest detectable glomerular change. Damage to this membrane and adjacent capillary wall cells permits leakage of proteins into the urine.

Natural history

- The progression of diabetic nephropathy towards end-stage renal failure proceeds through five stages.
  - ◇ Stage 1: Functional changes.
  - ◇ Stage 2: Structural changes.
  - ◇ Stage 3: Microalbuminuria.
  - ◇ Stage 4: Overt clinical nephropathy.
  - ◇ Stage 5: End-stage renal disease.
- After initial microalbuminuria, intraglomerular pressure is raised and finally, frank proteinuria develops with renal dysfunction (**114**).
- Diabetic nephropathy does not become symptomatic until renal dysfunction is severe.

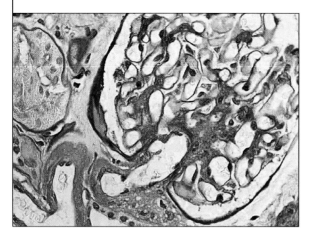

115 Early changes of diabetic nephropathy. There is mesangial expansion (pink-stained region), accompanied by basement membrane thickening. *Courtesy Barts and The London Hospital Trust.*

Stage 1: Functional changes

◆ Glomerular filtration rate (GFR) is increased due to an increase in intraglomerular pressure and in glomerular capillary surface area.

◆ The increase in GFR is related to the degree of hyperglycemia, and GFR usually falls as blood glucose levels improve, though it remains elevated in a proportion of patients.

◆ Serum creatinine can be decreased in this stage of hyperfiltration.

Stage 2: Structural changes

◆ Initially the glomerular basement membrane is thickened. The kidney is damaged such that the afferent arteriole (leading to the glomerulus) vasodilates more than the efferent glomerular arteriole.

◆ As a result the intraglomerular filtration pressure increases, further damaging the glomerular capillaries. Increased intraglomerular pressure causes increased shearing forces and increased secretion of extracellular mesangial matrix material (**115**). This process leads to glomerular hypertrophy, then sclerosis.

Stage 3: Microalbuminuria

◆ This is the earliest clinically detectable stage, and is sometimes called the stage of incipient diabetic nephropathy.

◆ Disruption of protein cross-linkages alters the glomerular filter, with progressive leakage of large molecules into the urine (**116**).

◇ Small quantities of albumin can be detected in the urine and can be estimated on a 24-h sample or more practically as an albumin/creatinine ratio from the first-voided urine sample (**117**).

116 Glomerular particle filtration. Rising glomerular pressure leads to loss of the negative charge on the glomerular basement membrane (GBM) and increases pore sizes. This consequently enables passage of plasma proteins, such as albumin and IgG, which is normally restricted.

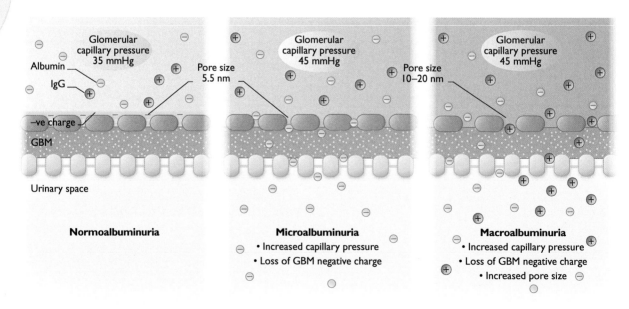

Microalbumin urine test

	SPOT URINE ALBUMIN/ CREATININE RATIO (mg/g)	24-HOUR URINARY ALBUMIN (mg/24 hr)	TIMED URINARY ALBUMIN EXCRETION (µg/min)
Normoalbuminuria	<30	<30	<20
Microalbuminuria	30–300	30–300	20–200
Macroalbuminuria	>300	>300	>200

Proteinuria is the hallmark of diabetic nephropathy.

◆ Microalbuminuria may be tested for by radio-immunoassay or by using sensitive dipsticks.

◆ It is a predictive marker of progression of nephropathy in type 1 diabetes (conferring a 20-fold increased risk of developing overt proteinuria or reduced GFR over 10 years), and less strongly in type 2 diabetes (5-fold increased risk over 10 years).

◆ It is a marker of macrovascular complications in both type 1 and type 2 diabetes.

◆ Left untreated, about 80% of type 1 diabetics with sustained microalbuminuria will progress to overt nephropathy in 10–15 years.

◆ Microalbuminuria worsens with uncontrolled glucose levels, elevated blood pressure, infections of the urinary tract, and exercise. It is therefore recommended to repeat testing for microalbuminuria when these conditions have resolved.

Stage 4: Overt clinical nephropathy

◆ As glomerular filtration falls, blood pressure and plasma creatinine rise, and proteinuria increases above 500 mg/day, but not usually to levels associated with the nephrotic syndrome.
◇ Urinary albumin excretion exceeds 300 mg/day.
◆ When overt nephropathy is left unattended in type 1 diabetes, GFR falls and end-stage renal disease (ESRD) develops in 50% of patients in 10 years, and about 75% in 20 years.
◆ Light-microscopic changes of glomerulosclerosis become manifest, both diffuse and nodular; the latter is known as the Kimmelstiel–Wilson node (**118**).

117 Definition of microalbuminuria. Microalbuminuria is defined as the excretion of between 30 and 300 mg of albumin a day in the urine.

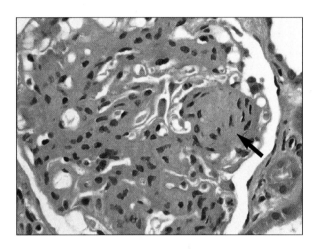

118 Late changes of diabetic glomerulosclerosis. More severe changes are apparent, with nodular lesions (arrow) within the mesangium, characterized by accumulation of homogeneous eosinophilic material (rounded acellular masses known as Kimmelstiel–Wilson nodes). *Courtesy Barts and The London Hospital Trust.*

Stage 5: End-stage renal disease
◆ Patients with ESRD typically show:
◇ Raised BUN.
◇ Raised creatinine.
◇ Decreased creatinine clearance.
◇ Anemia (normochromic normocytic).
◇ Altered calcium metabolism (low calcium, high phosphate).
◇ Dyslipidemia.
◇ Hypertension.

Diabetic kidney disease

Diagnosis of nephropathy

- ◆ Proteinuria is the hallmark of diabetic nephropathy.
- ◆ The urine of all diabetic patients should be checked for the presence of protein (**119**).
  - ◇ Screening for microalbuminuria is recommended annually for type 1 diabetic patients with diabetes duration of >5 years, and in type 2 patients at the time of diagnosis, since good glycemic control, early antihypertensive treatment, and the use of an ACEI at this stage may delay progression of nephropathy.

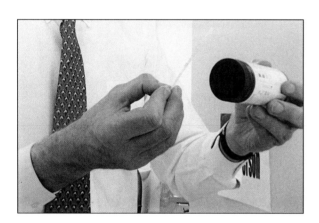

119 Urine strip testing for proteinuria. Persistent proteinuria is the hallmark of diabetic nephropathy; detection of hematuria suggests a different cause, such as menstruation, urinary tract infection, or vasculitis.

120 Differential diagnosis. There is a range of differentiating tests to exclude nondiabetic kidney disease.

Tests for nondiabetic causes of nephropathy

Urine microscopy for casts (vasculitis), red cells (nephritis), and culture (infection)

Serum protein electrophoresis (monoclonal bands = myeloma), calcium, phosphate, alkaline phosphatase, urate, ESR (raised ESR = myeloma or vasculitis), CRP

Serum for autoantibodies (vasculitis), including antinuclear autoantibodies and complement 4 levels

Renal ultrasound (large kidneys = polycystic; small kidneys = chronic pyelonephritis)

- ◆ Serum creatinine determination for estimation of the GFR is also recommended annually.
- ◆ There is no definitive test to verify that the nephropathy is due to diabetes, so other possible causes should be considered, including myeloma, autoimmune nephritis, and chronic pyelonephritis (**120**).
- ◆ Patients with diabetes can have renovascular disease leading to renal dysfunction, in which case they may not have proteinuria and are at risk of adverse responses to ACEIs. Renal biopsy might be considered to exclude a nondiabetic cause of nephropathy, but in practice it is rarely helpful or necessary.

Urinary tract infections

- ◆ Urinary tract infections are more common in diabetes. However, in well-controlled diabetes, some studies have not found a higher risk of infection compared to that in nondiabetic patients.
- ◆ Infections develop because of urinary stasis from autonomic neuropathy affecting bladder function or from impaired host defenses.
- ◆ Once a urinary tract infection develops, the complication rate is higher in diabetic than in nondiabetic patients, including the risk of pyelonephritis.
- ◆ Untreated infections in diabetic patients can lead to renal papillary necrosis, a rare condition in which renal papillae are shed in the urine. It should be suspected in patients who have fever, flank pain, poor response to antibiotics, and rapidly deteriorating renal function.

Treatment and management

- ◆ Management of diabetic nephropathy extends from the management of microalbuminuria to prevent disease progression through to the management of renal failure.
  - ◇ The management of diabetic nephropathy is similar to that of other causes of renal failure (**121**).
  - ◇ Particular attention must be paid to macrovascular risk factors and complications as well as the increased risk of neuropathy and retinopathy in patients with diabetic renal disease.

121 Diabetic kidney disease management in primary practice. Algorithm with routes to diagnosis, monitoring, and control. Control of hypertension and hyperglycemia is essential in patients with nephropathy. Angiotensin-converting enzyme inhibitors (ACEIs) and angiotensin-receptor blockers (ARBs) delay the progression of renal disease and have antiproteinuric and renoprotective effects.

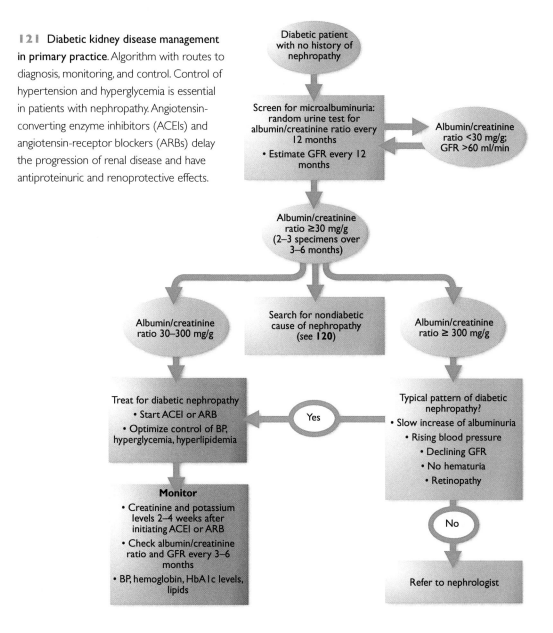

Look out for macrovascular risk factors in patients with diabetic renal disease.

General therapy

◆ Once renal dysfunction has been established therapy should include:
  ◇ Phosphate binders such as calcium carbonate.
  ◇ Vitamin D analogs once serum parathyroid hormone increases.
  ◇ Erythropoietin once hemoglobin falls significantly.
  ◇ Multivitamins.
  ◇ Antacids such as ranitidine.

Blood glucose

◆ Intensive glucose control is helpful in the earlier stages of renal involvement (**122**):
  ◇ In the DCCT, intensive glycemic control in type 1 diabetes patients reduced the occurrence of microalbuminuria by 39%, and of overt proteinuria by 54% (**123**).
  ◇ In the UKPDS intensive glycemic control led to a 30% reduction in microalbuminuria risk.
  ◇ In the Steno-2 study there was a 61% reduction in progression to clinical nephropathy with intervention directed at glucose, lipids, and blood pressure.

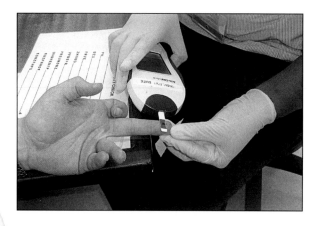

122 Capillary blood glucose measurement. Optimal glycemic control is helpful in the early stages of kidney disease.

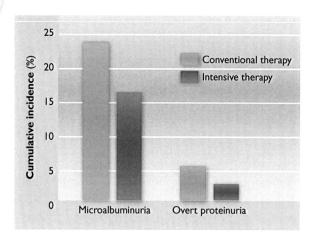

123 Nephropathy event rates. The DCCT showed that stringent glycemic control dramatically reduced the risk of developing diabetic nephropathy.

◆ Therapy should aim to achieve an HbA1c of <7.0% (53 mmol/mol) or <6.5% (48 mmol/mol) (in the US) without causing severe hypoglycemia.
◆ However, the initiation of intensive glucose control after the onset of overt proteinuria or renal insufficiency is often ineffective in preventing progression to ESRD.
◆ Once the creatinine has risen to 130 µmol/l (1.5 mg/dl) metformin should not be used, while the dose of other agents should be monitored carefully.

Blood pressure

◆ Tight control and aggressive treatment of blood pressure (target 130/80 mmHg) reduce the rate of progression to renal failure (**124**).
◆ In patients with nephropathy, it can be argued that ACEIs and ARBs are preferred.
◆ ACEIs are specifically indicated in type 1 diabetes where there is any degree of albuminuria (with or without hypertension).
◆ ARBs have a role when there is intolerance to ACEIs, and are the drug class recommended in patients with type 2 diabetes, hypertension, and any degree of albuminuria.
  ◇ In type 2 diabetes with hypertension and nephropathy, ARBs prevented the progression of microalbuminuria to overt nephropathy in the Irbesartan in Patients with Type 2 Diabetes and Microalbuminuria (IRMA-2) study (**125**).
  ◇ ARBs also reduced the incidence of doubling of serum creatinine and the risk of developing ESRD in those who had later stages of nephropathy in the Irbesartan Type 2 Diabetic Nephropathy Trial (IDNT) and Reduction of Endpoints in NIDDM with the Angiotensin II Antagonist Losartan (RENAAL) Trial.
◆ Combining ACEIs with calcium-channel blockers or thiazide diuretics may provide superior blood pressure control.
◆ Loop diuretics are used in preference to thiazides once nephropathy is established, usually around a serum creatinine of 160 µmol/l (1.8 mg/dl).
◆ Combination therapy is usually required to achieve the blood pressure target.

Diabetic kidney disease

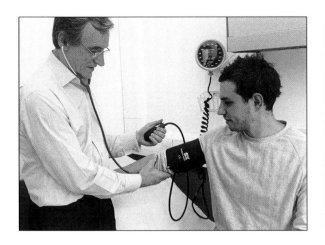

124 Blood pressure measurement. Control of hypertension reduces the rate of progression to renal failure.

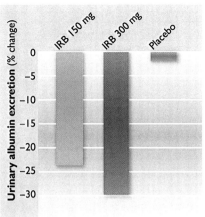

125 Irbesartan in patients with diabetes and micro-albuminuria. The IRMA-2 study showed that patients receiving daily irbesartan were significantly less likely to develop diabetic nephropathy than those in the placebo group.

◆ Beta-adrenoreceptor blockers should be considered in all patients with coronary artery disease and in patients after a myocardial infarction, since these agents improve survival.
  ◇ The beta-blocker atenolol reduced microvascular complications in diabetic patients in the UKPDS.
  ◇ However, beta-blockers are third-line treatment in the management of hypertension in diabetes – certainly for type 2 diabetes. For example, the ARB losartan reduced cardiovascular mortality more than did atenolol in patients with diabetes and hypertension in the Losartan Intervention for Endpoint Reduction (LIFE) study (adjusted risk reduction of 13% after 66 months).
  ◇ Patients taking insulin therapy should be careful as beta-adrenergic blocking agents may mask some epinephrine-induced symptoms of hypoglycemia, though sweating may be more pronounced.

Lipids
◆ Once proteinuria is established, the risk of macrovascular disease is sufficient to warrant use of statins, if the patient is not already on them. Even if the usual picture of dyslipidemia in diabetes is that of hypertriglyceridemia, low HDL-cholesterol, and LDL-cholesterol that is within normal levels, elevated LDL-cholesterol is common in patients with marked proteinuria.

◆ Mortality in patients with ESRD is usually cardiovascular in nature.
◆ Treatment with statins at high dose (or less commonly and debatably statins with fibrates) is often needed to achieve targets: LDL-cholesterol <2.59 mmol/l (100 mg/dl), triglycerides <1.7 mmol/l (150 mg/dl) and HDL-cholesterol to 1.17 mmol/l (45 mg/dl).
◆ The risk of myositis is increased in renal impairment when cyclosporins plus statins or fibrates are used, and other pharmacological agents may have to be substituted.

Smoking
◆ Smoking predisposes to diabetic nephropathy and should be particularly avoided once nephropathy is established due to the risk of macrovascular disease.

Protein restriction
◆ A reduction in protein intake reduces hyperfiltration, intraglomerular pressure, and proteinuria.
◆ Earlier studies showed that very low-protein diets slowed down the decline in GFR, however, with the advent of antihypertensive and renoprotective agents such as ACEIs, it seems that modest protein restriction at 1.0 g/kg/day is appropriate.

Diabetic kidney disease

Renal replacement therapy

- ◆ Once the creatinine rises, in association with deteriorating creatinine clearance and GFR, referral to renal physicians is appropriate, and if above 500 μmol/l (5.65 mg/dl) (depending on local guidelines) renal replacement should be considered, especially if symptoms develop.
- ◆ Plotting the inverse of creatinine against time gives an indication as to the rate of progression of renal dysfunction so that renal replacement can be planned in advance (**126**).
- ◆ There are three forms of renal replacement:
  - ◇ Continuous ambulatory peritoneal dialysis (CAPD).
  - ◇ Hemodialysis.
  - ◇ Transplantation.

In 2005, a total of 178,689 people in the USA and Puerto Rico with ESRD due to diabetes were living on chronic dialysis or with a kidney transplant.

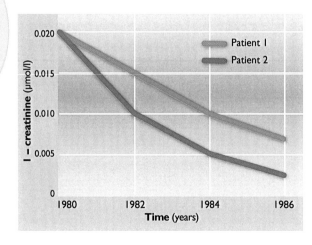

126 Progression of renal dysfunction. Once GFR has fallen by 50% or more, serum creatinine begins to increase. Plots of inverse creatinine against time in two type 1 diabetes patients, each 15 years from diagnosis, with persistent proteinuria, show a linear decline at a consistent rate for each patient.

Continuous ambulatory peritoneal dialysis

- ◆ Management of ESRD is made more difficult by the fact that patients often have other complications of diabetes such as blindness, autonomic neuropathy, or peripheral vascular disease. Vascular shunts tend to calcify rapidly and hence CAPD may be preferable to hemodialysis. However, in some countries such as the US where many dialysis centers are available, or where there are barriers to self-care, hemodialysis seems to be the more common modality.
- ◆ CAPD is inexpensive compared with the other replacement therapies and avoids fluctuations in intravascular volume, a problem seen in patients with cardiac disease or autonomic neuropathy. Vascular access is not required.
- ◆ This form of dialysis provides greater mobility for the patient compared to hemodialysis.
- ◆ The dialysate contains hypertonic glucose, and since the dialysis is a continuous process, hyperglycemia is a problem. To address this, insulin is usually added to the dialysis and is delivered intraperitoneally.
- ◆ Peritonitis is a complication seen with CAPD.

Hemodialysis

- ◆ Hemodialysis is the renal replacement used in 80% of diabetic patients with ESRD in the US.
- ◆ Hemodialysis requires vascular access, usually an arteriovenous fistula. Because of problems with calcification and atherosclerosis, a synthetic graft is sometimes needed.
  - ◇ Vascular access should be established sooner than in nondiabetic patients since retinopathy, neuropathy, hypertension, and glycemic control become more difficult to manage when diabetic patients have uremia.
  - ◇ At a serum creatinine of 265–354 μmol/l (3–4 mg/dl), a rapid decline in kidney function ensues in diabetic patients such that dialysis is needed in less than a year.
- ◆ Hemodialysis is more prone to induce hypotension than is CAPD.
- ◆ Necrosis of digits can be a particular problem.

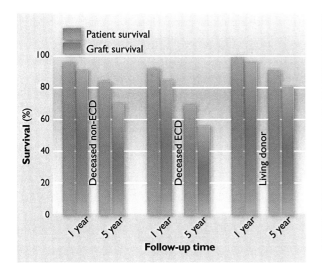

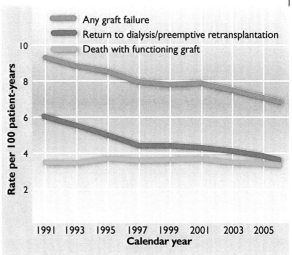

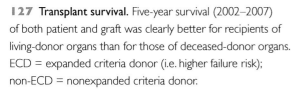

127 Transplant survival. Five-year survival (2002–2007) of both patient and graft was clearly better for recipients of living-donor organs than for those of deceased-donor organs. ECD = expanded criteria donor (i.e. higher failure risk); non-ECD = nonexpanded criteria donor.

128 Transplant failure rates. These have gradually improved. In the USA, by 2006 there were 6.9 graft failures (including death with function) per 100 patient-years with a functioning transplant.

Transplantation

◆ Renal transplant involves obtaining the kidney from a cadaver or, less frequently, from a living-related or living-unrelated donor.

◆ Patient survival is superior compared to dialysis. In diabetes both patient survival and graft survival are slightly reduced compared with nondiabetic patients.

◆ Assessment of the patient to exclude life-limiting comorbidity, including macrovascular disease, is vital before a transplant is performed.

◆ Cardiovascular disease is still the most common cause of death in patients who undergo transplantation.

◆ Graft and patient survival have improved with time for both living-donor and cadaveric transplants, but is still better with living-donor compared with nonexpanded criteria (deceased) donors (non-ECD) and expanded criteria (deceased) donors (ECD) (**127, 128**).

◇ ECD refers to donors with a higher risk of kidney graft failure, such as donors who are over 60 years old, or aged more than 50 years with at least two of the following: hypertension history, serum creatinine >132.6 µmol/l (1.5 mg/dl), or cause of death from cerebrovascular accident.

Pancreas transplant or islet cell implantation

◆ A segmental pancreatic graft is sometimes performed at the same time as a renal graft. Although pancreatic transplants have a limited viability, owing to progressive fibrosis within the graft, they may give the patient a year or so of freedom from insulin injections.

◆ There has been interest in islet cell implants, which currently have a limited role in the management of diabetes.

◇ The limited role stems from the limited success in achieving insulin treatment independence in patients allied to the use of drugs to reduce the immune response with potentially serious side-effects, including cancer risk.

◇ Indications for treatment are confined to those patients with type 1 diabetes who are not children or in old age and who experience prolonged and severe lifestyle restrictions owing to impaired warning of hypoglycemia.

CHAPTER 11

Severe diabetic metabolic disturbances

Diabetic ketoacidosis

◆ Metabolic disturbances in diabetes can have extremely serious consequences. If unrecognized, they may result in coma.

◆ Diabetic ketoacidosis (DKA) is a life-threatening condition that can be reversed if there is early recognition and prompt treatment.

◆ The underlying pathology is insulin deficiency, leading to blood glucose generally >13.9 mmol/l (250 mg/dl), pH <7.3, and a bicarbonate of usually <15 mmol/l (15 mEq/l).

◆ Most of the time it is easy to differentiate between DKA and hyperosmolar nonketotic hyperglycemia (HONK – see p. 128), but in some situations features may overlap (**129**).

◆ Diabetic ketoacidosis is often precipitated by:
  ◇ Omission of insulin.
  ◇ Infection.
  ◇ Myocardial infarction.
  ◇ Trauma.

◆ DKA in people under the age of 25 is rarely attributable to infection or other intercurrent illness; it is most probably due to patient noncompliance, e.g. stopping insulin, excess alcohol, or recreational drug use.

◆ Ketoacidosis is predominantly seen in type 1 diabetes.
  ◇ It can also occur in type 2 diabetes under stressful conditions such as infections, myocardial infarction, trauma; it may be induced by atypical antipsychotic agents such as risperidone and olanzepine.

◆ DKA is the presentation at diagnosis in 20–25% of type 1 diabetes patients.
  ◇ The majority of DKA episodes occur in previously known rather than newly diagnosed diabetes.
  ◇ About 20% of patients who have had DKA have multiple episodes in a year.

◆ The majority of cases reaching hospital are preventable because the metabolic disturbances take a while to develop and often result from the patient being unaware of how to manage insulin therapy. Important components of prevention therefore include:
  ◇ Earlier detection.
  ◇ Proper education.
  ◇ Good communication between patient and physician.
  ◇ The capacity to self-manage insulin injections at home even when sick. Sick-day rules should be part of the education given to patients so that they may give themselves bolus doses of insulin while awaiting further instructions from their physician.

Comparison of DKA and HONK

DKA	HONK
Hyperketonemia	No hyperketonemia
Metabolic acidosis	Metabolic acidosis in some cases
Severe hyperglycemia	Severe hyperglycemia

129 Features of DKA and HONK. The main distinguishing feature of DKA is the presence of significant ketoacidosis.

122

- For patients on an insulin pump, detachment and malfunction of the pump and delivery system can be readily suspected with rising glucose levels on frequent capillary blood glucose checks, thereby alerting the patient to take steps to avert DKA. It is important to realize that DKA will develop rapidly, within several hours, in a patient treated with a subcutaneous insulin infusion pump in the event of pump failure, due to the lack of any depot of long-acting insulin.
- In about one quarter of DKA cases the patients reduced or omitted their insulin doses because they were not eating due to nausea or vomiting. In this situation insulin needs to be increased, not reduced. This strengthens the case that continued education needs to be provided to patients, their family, and friends. Insulin should never be stopped without medical advice.

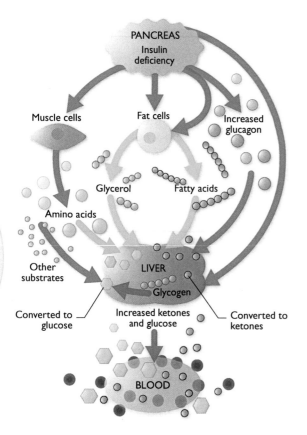

130 Pathogenesis of diabetic ketoacidosis. Insulin deficiency and the concomitant increase in glucagon lead to increased breakdown of triglycerides into free fatty acids, and increased hepatic glycogenolysis, gluconeogenesis, and ketogenesis.

Education about managing insulin therapy is essential in the prevention of DKA.

Pathogenesis
- Ketoacidosis is the primary manifestation, and results from a deficiency of insulin and the resulting uncontrolled catabolism from excess counter-regulatory hormones – glucagon, epinephrine, cortisol, and growth hormone (see also p. 34).
  - ◇ Only modest insulin levels are needed to inhibit hepatic ketogenesis, so when there is absolute or relative insulin deficiency, ketogenesis ensues.
  - ◇ As ketoacids are produced, bicarbonate and other buffers are lost, and metabolic acidosis follows.
  - ◇ With insulin deficiency, glucagon stimulates gluconeogenesis and ketogenesis. As the other counter-regulatory hormones come into play, peripheral glucose utilization is inhibited, and lipolysis takes place (**130**).
- After ketoacidosis, the second important feature is fluid depletion resulting from diuresis (**131**).
  - ◇ The blood glucose may be 10–20 mmol/l (180–360 mg/dl) in some cases, particularly in children, but is usually in excess of 20 mmol/l (360 mg/dl).
  - ◇ Glycosuria results as blood glucose levels exceed the renal threshold. Hyperglycemia causes an osmotic diuresis, with loss of both water and electrolytes.
- Ketoacidosis and fluid depletion occurring together exacerbate the condition through a fall in muscle and renal perfusion. The excess of glucagon and epinephrine exacerbates the insulin deficiency and results in additional metabolic derangement, e.g. increased lipolysis and ketone body production, the latter predisposing to vomiting.
- Rapid lipolysis occurs, leading to elevated circulating free fatty acid levels. The free fatty acids are broken down to fatty acyl-CoA within the liver cells, and this in turn is converted to ketone bodies within the mitochondria.
  - ◇ Accumulation of ketone bodies leads to metabolic acidosis.

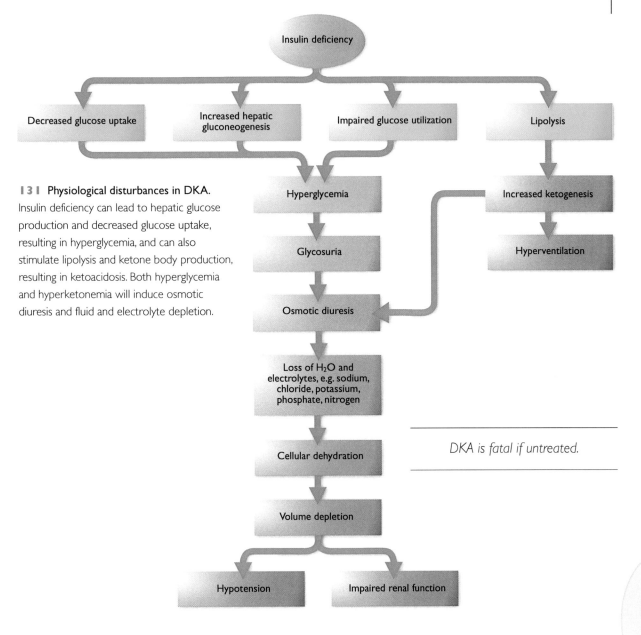

131 Physiological disturbances in DKA.
Insulin deficiency can lead to hepatic glucose
production and decreased glucose uptake,
resulting in hyperglycemia, and can also
stimulate lipolysis and ketone body production,
resulting in ketoacidosis. Both hyperglycemia
and hyperketonemia will induce osmotic
diuresis and fluid and electrolyte depletion.

Insulin deficiency

Decreased glucose uptake

Increased hepatic gluconeogenesis

Impaired glucose utilization

Lipolysis

Hyperglycemia

Increased ketogenesis

Glycosuria

Hyperventilation

Osmotic diuresis

Loss of H_2O and electrolytes, e.g. sodium, chloride, potassium, phosphate, nitrogen

DKA is fatal if untreated.

Cellular dehydration

Volume depletion

Hypotension

Impaired renal function

◆ Vomiting exacerbates loss of fluid and electrolytes.
◆ The excess ketones are excreted in the urine but
also appear in the breath, producing a distinctive
smell similar to that of acetone.
◆ Respiratory compensation for the acidosis leads
to hyperventilation, described as 'air hunger'.
◆ Progressive dehydration impairs renal excretion
of hydrogen ions and ketones, which are
retained, aggravating the acidosis.

◆ As the pH falls below 7.0 ([H⁺] >100 nmol/l), pH-
dependent enzyme systems in many cells
function less effectively.
◆ Untreated DKA is invariably fatal.
  ◇ In tertiary centers, the mortality rate is <5%.
  ◇ The highest mortality occurs in patients aged
  75 years or older.
  ◇ In children, cerebral edema is a complication
  that increases the risk of mortality.
  ◇ Coma as a presenting sign also carries a high
  risk of mortality.

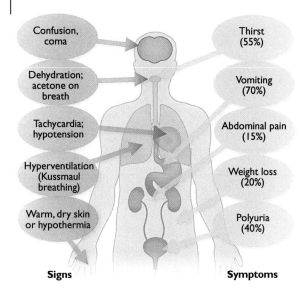

Signs   **Symptoms**

132 Clinical features of ketoacidosis. Normally DKA has a rapid onset, but some symptoms, such as weight loss and lethargy, may develop several weeks before presentation.

Clinical features
◆ Clinically a patient with diabetic ketoacidosis is very unwell, even comatose, with marked weight loss, thirst, and polyuria. They may be gasping for air or vomiting (**132**).

Investigations
◆ The initial investigations to be done in suspected DKA include blood and urine tests, bacteriology, ECG, and imaging (**133**).
  ◇ It is important to differentiate DKA from other causes of coma or altered consciousness (**134**).
◆ DKA often results in high anion gap acidosis, with the 'gap' being the unmeasured anions in the plasma, primarily albumin and phosphate.
  ◇ Anion gap (in mEq/l or mmol/l) is measured as:
    Measured (or uncorrected) serum sodium – (chloride + bicarbonate).
  ◇ A value of 12 mmol/l (mEq/l) is usually taken as the cut-off to determine if the anion gap is increased.

134 Coma and impaired consciousness. A decrease in the level of consciousness may be attributable to causes other than DKA.

Initial investigations in ketoacidosis

Blood	Glucose, creatinine and electrolytes, full blood count, arterial blood gases including pH, blood ketones, beta-hydroxybutyrate, blood culture
Urine	Dipstick analysis for ketones, pyuria, blood, protein, and urine culture
Bacteriology	Swab any infection and as above do blood and urine cultures
ECG	To detect peaked T waves (hyperkalemia), flat T waves (hypokalemia), or undetected arrhythmia or infarction
Chest radiography	To detect infection or cardiac failure
CT or MRI scan	If cerebral edema is suspected or cause of coma unclear
Other investigations	Directed at finding the precipitating cause

133 Investigations. Glucose and blood gas measurements should be obtained without delay.

Other causes of coma or impaired consciousness

Hyperosmolar nonketotic coma

Hypoglycemia

Other electrolyte disorders such as hyponatremia, hypernatremia, hypercalcemia

Head trauma

Toxins, drugs

Uremia

Lactic acidosis

Hepatic encephalopathy

Hypoxemia

CNS infections

Intracranial lesions such as hemorrhage, stroke, hematoma, abscess

- Other causes of high anion gap acidosis are usually easy to distinguish from DKA, but should be kept in mind if the presentation is not straightforward.
  - ◇ Salicylate poisoning can be tested by plasma salicylate levels in the toxic range.
  - ◇ Ethylene glycol or methanol poisoning is suspected if there is an 'osmolal gap', i.e. the measured plasma osmolality is greater than the calculated plasma osmolality.
  - ◇ Alcoholic acidosis and starvation acidosis also present with increased anion gap.

Acute management

- The principles of management in adult patients are given below. Children will require different proportions and volumes.
- *Fluid.* Fluid replacement must be started immediately.
  - ◇ Normal saline is given at an initial rate of 1 l/hr, or 15–20 ml/kg/hr for the first 1–2 hr. Careful monitoring should be done when treating patients at risk of cardiovascular disease and cardiac or renal dysfunction.
  - ◇ Thereafter, fluids can be reduced to 4–14 ml/kg/hr using normal saline or (controversially) 0.45% saline depending on the patient's sodium level and state of hydration.
- *Insulin deficiency.* An initial dose of regular insulin, 0.15 U/kg, can be given as an intravenous bolus. Afterwards, regular insulin intravenous infusion is given at 5–10 U/hr or at 0.1 U/kg/hr.
  - ◇ This lowers blood glucose by suppressing hepatic glucose output.
  - ◇ Regular insulin, 50 U, can be added to 500 ml of normal saline to make a 1:10 concentration. Some of the solution is then flushed to prime the tubing.
  - ◇ In some instances, the intramuscular route can be used at an initial dose of 0.5 U/kg, then hourly at a dose of 0.1 U/kg/hr.
  - ◇ The subcutaneous route is usually avoided because subcutaneous blood flow is reduced in shocked patients and insulin action is slower.
- *Electrolytes.* Potassium levels must be monitored both with blood tests and by ECG.
  - ◇ Although there is a total body potassium deficit, initially potassium in the blood may be high.

- ◇ If initial serum K⁺ is 5.0 mmol/l (mEq/l), replacement is not given and K⁺ levels are checked every 2 hr.
- ◇ When K⁺ is in the normal range (3.5–5.0 mmol/l [mEq/l]), 20–30 mmol/l [mEq] K⁺ is given in each liter of intravenous fluid.
- ◇ If K⁺ is less than 3.3 mmol/l (mEq/l), insulin is withheld until K⁺ is above 3.5 mmol/l (mEq/l) and K⁺ is given at 40 mmol/l/hr (mEq/l/hr).
- *Acid–base balance.* Both fluid replacement and insulin therapy will usually restore acid–base imbalance.
  - ◇ Administration of bicarbonate is controversial and seldom necessary and is only considered if the pH is below 7.0 ([H⁺] >100 nmol/l); if given, bicarbonate is best administered as an isotonic (1.35%) solution, if available.
  - ◇ Prospective studies have not shown either a benefit or an increased morbidity or mortality in patients where pH is 6.9–7.1. Below a pH of 7.0, even in the absence of solid data, it seems reasonable to administer bicarbonate since severe acidosis can also lead to vascular derangements.
- Successful management of DKA depends upon fluid resuscitation, insulin therapy, and correcting metabolic acidosis and electrolyte imbalances. Frequent monitoring of these parameters is necessary (**135**). A treatment algorithm (**136**) is given overleaf.

Initial monitoring interval for DKA parameters

Vital signs and mental status	Every hour
Glucose	Every hour
Potassium	Every 2 hours
Other electrolytes, blood urea nitrogen (BUN), creatinine	Every 4 hours

135 Monitoring. Regular, frequent monitoring is required to assess progress and avoid complications.

Severe diabetic metabolic disturbances

DIABETIC KETOACIDOSIS

Complete initial evaluation.
Check capillary glucose and serum/urine ketones
to confirm hyperglycemia and ketonemia/ketonuria.
Start IV fluids (1.0 l/hr of 0.9% NaCl initially)

IV fluids | **Insulin** | **Potassium** | **Bicarbonate**

IV fluids
• Determine hydration status

Insulin
• Give IV insulin infusion (0.1 U/kg/hr)

Potassium
• If serum K$^+$ level is <3.3 mmol/l, withhold insulin and give K$^+$ (40 mmol/l IV) until >3.5 mmol/l

Bicarbonate
• Rarely used
• After 1 hr of hydration, check pH

Hypovolemic shock | Mild hypotension | Cardiogenic shock

pH <7 | pH ≥7

• Check serum glucose every hour
• If level does not fall by <3 mmol/l within 1 hr then double insulin dose

• If serum K$^+$ level is ≥5 mmol/l, withhold K$^+$
• Check K$^+$ level every 2 hr

• 0.9% NaCl (1.0 l/hr) or plasma expanders, or both

• Evaluate corrected serum Na$^+$ level

• Hemodynamic monitoring

• Dilute NaHCO$_3$ (50 mmol) in 200 ml sterile H$_2$O
• Infuse at a rate of 200 ml/hr

• No NaHCO$_3$

High Na$^+$ | Normal Na$^+$ | Low Na$^+$

• If serum K$^+$ level is 3.3–5.0 mmol/l, give K$^+$ (20 mmol/l IV) to maintain at 4–5 mmol/l

• Repeat NaHCO$_3$ every 2 hr until pH >7.0
• Monitor serum K$^+$ level

• 0.45% NaCl (4–14 ml/kg hr) depending on hydration status

• 0.9% NaCl (4–14 ml/kg hr) depending on hydration status

• Once blood glucose is 12–14 mmol/l, switch to 5% dextrose with 0.45% NaCl and reduce insulin infusion to 0.05–0.1 U/kg/hr

• Once clinically stable, start subcutaneous insulin regime; continue IV insulin for 2–4 hr after initiation of SC insulin
• Look for precipitating causes

• Check electrolytes, BUN, venous pH, creatinine, and glucose every 2–4 hr until stable

Severe diabetic metabolic disturbances

136 Treatment algorithm for DKA in adults. The corner-stones of acute management are fluid resuscitation, insulin therapy, correction of metabolic acidosis and electrolyte abnormalities, as well as treatment of precipitating factors.

◆ ***Seek the underlying cause.*** Physical examination, chest radiography, and urine tests may reveal a source of infection.
  ◇ As fever may be absent even in the presence of infection, and polymorpholeukocytosis can be present even in the absence of infection, a search for other causes can be directed by the patient's clinical features.
  ◇ For example, a 65-year-old male with hypertension and positive smoking history would lead you to obtain an ECG to exclude a silent myocardial infarction, which can present with ketoacidosis.
◆ ***Other problems.*** These can include:
  ◇ Altered sensorium. For patients in coma, the insertion of a nasogastric tube can help reduce the risk of aspiration pneumonia.
  ◇ Hypotension. Intravenous fluid resuscitation should be administered. If hypotension continues, plasma expanders or whole blood may be considered, as well as insertion of a central venous pressure line.
  ◇ Hypothermia. Mortality rate is high, about 30–60%, in patients with DKA and hypothermia.
  ◇ Cerebral edema. This is most often seen in children and adolescents. The cause is thought to be very rapid correction of hyperglycemia and the use of excessive hypotonic fluids. Though rare, it can be fatal.
  ◇ Deep venous thrombosis can be prevented by prophylactic measures such as subcutaneous heparin.
  ◇ Complications of therapy. With excess insulin infusion, hypoglycemia and hypokalemia can develop, hence the need for close monitoring of these parameters. Excess fluid replacement can cause cardiac dysfunction; in patients with cardiac compromise, monitoring of central venous pressure is recommended.

Subsequent management

◆ Once glucose reaches 13 mmol/l (235 mg/dl), the infusion is changed to 5% dextrose in 0.45% NaCl at 150–250 ml/hr until acidosis is corrected. The addition of dextrose allows continued infusion of insulin without hypoglycemia, since it takes longer to clear the acidosis than to lower the blood glucose.
◆ When the acidosis has been corrected, insulin is then given through the subcutaneous route.
  ◇ The intravenous insulin infusion is turned off 2–4 hours after the first subcutaneous dose of insulin is given, depending on the kind of subcutaneous insulin used. The insulin infusion is not discontinued right away since the half-life of intravenous insulin is just a few minutes.
◆ Once the patient is able to eat, the dextrose infusion can be taken down.
◆ One subcutaneous insulin regimen that closely mimics the physiological secretion of insulin by the pancreas is the administration of long-acting insulin such as glargine once a day (occasionally even twice daily) or detemir, with rapid-acting insulin such as lispro or aspart or glulisine before meals.
◆ The total daily dose of subcutaneous insulin can be determined in three ways. Using a combination of these methods is helpful to make sure an appropriate dose is arrived at:
  ◇ Estimation of the dose required via the intravenous insulin infusion (calculate requirements from the past 6 or 8 hours and multiply by 4 or 3, respectively, to come up with a 24-hour dose).
  ◇ Basing it on total body weight. 0.3 U/kg/day is usually a good dose for newly diagnosed diabetics; the dose increases if the duration of diabetes is longer, or if the patient has features of insulin resistance.
  ◇ Basing it on home insulin doses and adjusting for degree of control prior to the episode of DKA.

Monitoring of glucose, potassium, and fluid levels is essential in order to avoid complications of therapy.

Severe diabetic metabolic disturbances

◆ Sliding-scale regimens have been popularized, but these reflect lack of familiarity with insulin dosage and may delay the establishment of stable blood glucose levels.

◇ Sliding scales are reactive and not proactive; rapid-acting or short-acting insulin is usually just given when blood glucoses are elevated, and insulin is omitted when blood glucoses are within the normal range. Basal insulin is not provided. Unfortunately, sliding scales have permeated the medical culture, for they ensure that the house staff get called only when blood glucose levels are too high or too low.

◇ Re-education of medical providers is needed so that basal and prandial insulin are administered.

◆ For patients who were on an insulin pump prior to the episode of DKA, proper functioning of the entire pump system has to be ascertained prior to resuming its use, since clogging and failure of insulin delivery are potential causes of DKA.

◆ Confirmation of the cause of DKA with a review of the history and investigations is important so that patients can be advised on how to avoid its recurrence.

A thorough search for the precipitating cause of HONK is essential.

---

137 HONK: precipitating factors. Common precipitating factors are infection and inadequate insulin therapy. Underlying medical conditions, particularly in the elderly, can lead to reduced water intake and the development of severe dehydration.

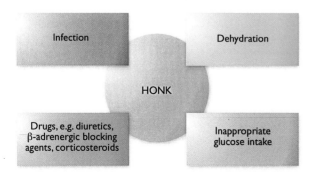

Hyperosmolar nonketotic hyperglycemia

◆ Hyperosmolar nonketotic hyperglycemia (HONK) is also known as hyperosmolar hyperglycemic state (HHS), hyperosmolar nonketotic state, and hyperosmolar nonketotic coma.

◆ HONK is characterized by severe hyperglycemia, dehydration, hyperosmolality, and absence of significant ketoacidosis.

◆ These patients usually have type 2 diabetes, so patients are often adults; however it can also occur in type 1 diabetic patients.

◆ Blood glucose is generally higher than in DKA, reaching levels of 33 mmol/l (600 mg/dl) or more, and sometimes greater than 83 mmol/l (1500 mg/dl), with a serum osmolality greater than 320 mmol/l (mOsm/kg).

◆ High anion gap acidosis is not normally found, but patients can have acidosis from poor tissue perfusion (lactic acidosis), uremia, and from ketone formation.

◆ As with DKA, an underlying illness must be sought. Common precipitating factors (**137**) causing HONK include:

◇ Intercurrent illness (such as infection, trauma, myocardial infarction).

◇ Medications such as steroids or thiazide diuretics.

◇ Drinking glucose-rich or 'energy' drinks. In patients who are not able to achieve adequate hydration, osmotic diuresis from the glucosuria and impaired concentrating ability of the kidneys lead to further rises in glucose levels.

◆ HONK and DKA represent two ends of a common spectrum (**138**). Severe cases are easily distinguishable from each other, but milder cases may be less distinct. The biochemical differences between the two conditions are due to:

◇ *Age.* Severe dehydration seen in HONK may be due to altered thirst (caused by an impaired cerebral thirst center) leading to less impetus to access fluids. The same problem can arise from restricted access to fluids (e.g. from physical disability, mental deficiency).

◇ *Degree of insulin deficiency.* In type 2 diabetes, though there is relative lack of insulin, there is often enough endogenous insulin to inhibit ketogenesis.

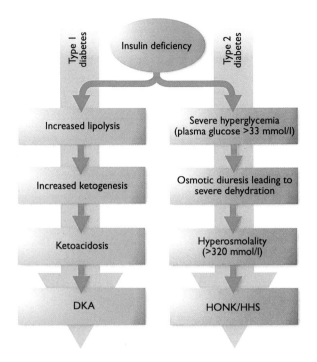

138 HONK and DKA. HONK differs clinically from DKA by an absence of ketoacidosis and a higher degree of hyperglycemia. It is further characterized by high osmolality and dehydration. HONK will often present in a patient with previously undiagnosed type 2 diabetes.

- The measured serum sodium is often falsely low because of the osmotic effect of glucose. To calculate for corrected serum sodium, 1.6 mmol/l (mEq) of Na^+ is added for each 5.5 mmol/l (100 mg/dl) of glucose above 5.5 mmol/l (100 mg/dl) or:
  - ◇ Corrected serum Na in mEq/l = measured Na in mEq/l + (1.6 [glucose in mg/dl – 100] divided by 100). If using glucose in mmol/l, multiply glucose by 18 first.
- Blood glucose should be checked hourly.
- HONK patients are usually older than patients who have DKA and mortality is higher, so a thorough search for the precipitating cause is important and will direct further management.
  - ◇ Chest radiography, urinalysis and cultures to look for infection, and an ECG to rule out myocardial infarction are reasonable screening tests, especially if a good history is unobtainable and physical findings are lacking.
  - ◇ In patients presenting with altered mental status, a stroke or an intracranial bleed should be considered.

Clinical features

- Typically patients are over 60 years of age, often with previously undiagnosed type 2 diabetes. A history of diuretic or steroid therapy is an additional risk factor.
- The history often is that of days to weeks of increasing thirst and polyuria, with weight loss and weakness.
- On presentation, patients have severe dehydration and altered mentation. Impairment of consciousness is related to the degree of hyperosmolality.
  - ◇ Abdominal complaints such as nausea and vomiting are not as common as in DKA.
- On examination, patients have poor skin turgor, hypotension, and tachycardia. Kussmaul breathing is uncommon.

Investigations

- Serum osmolality is usually greater than 320 mmol/l (mOsm/kg), and glucose greater than 33 mmol/l (600 mg/dl). Serum osmolality is measured as:
  2 [Na + K (in mmol/l or mEq/l)] + blood glucose (divided by 1 when using mmol/l, or by 18 when using glucose in mg/dl).
- Monitoring of serum osmolality and electrolytes is key to management, and should be checked every 2–4 hours.

Complications

- Vascular occlusions are important complications of HONK.
  - ◇ Arterial thrombosis is said to cause one third of the deaths in diabetic coma. Arterial thrombosis leads to cerebrovascular accidents, myocardial infarction, or arterial insufficiency in the lower limbs.
  - ◇ Mesenteric artery occlusion and disseminated intravascular coagulation may also occur.

Patients with HONK are particularly prone to arterial thrombosis.

Severe diabetic metabolic disturbances

Treatment

- The general principles of management are similar to those for DKA. However, the following are the differences or points of emphasis:
  - ◇ Plasma osmolality is often very high. This should be monitored as treatment progresses. Normal osmolality is between 280 and 295 mmol/l or mOsm/kg.
  - ◇ Normal saline is recommended for fluid replacement. Half-normal saline (0.45%) may result in rapid hemodilution and subsequent cerebral damage.
  - ◇ Patients can be sensitive to insulin. With a brisk fall in glucose, smaller insulin doses (e.g. 3 U/hr not 6 U/hr) are appropriate. Otherwise, a rapid fall in glucose may result in cerebral edema.
  - ◇ Anticoagulant prophylaxis is particularly important.

Prognosis

- Mortality in HONK is seen in 10–50% of cases, on the higher end for the elderly.
- For patients who recover, however, many can be treated with diet and oral agents alone.

Brittle diabetes mellitus

- This term is used to describe patients with recurrent ketoacidosis and/or recurrent hypoglycemic coma, but there is no precise definition. Most patients are those who experience recurrent severe hypoglycemia.
  - ◇ It has been said that there is no such thing as brittle diabetes only brittle diabetics.
- Once underlying causes and improvements in management have been implemented attention should focus on psychosocial issues.

Recurrent ketoacidosis

- This usually occurs in adolescents or young adults, particularly girls. Metabolic decompensation may develop very rapidly.
- A combination of chaotic food intake and insulin omission, whether consciously or unconsciously, is now regarded as the primary cause of this problem. It almost always occurs in the context of considerable psychosocial problems, particularly eating disorders. This area needs careful and sympathetic exploration in any patient with recurrent ketoacidosis. It is perhaps not surprising that in an illness where much of one's life is spent thinking of and controlling food intake, 30% of women with diabetes have had some features of an eating disorder at some time.
- Other causes include:
  - ◇ Iatrogenic. Inappropriate insulin combinations may be a cause of swinging glycemic control. For example, a once-daily regimen may cause hypoglycemia during the afternoon or evening and pre-breakfast hyperglycemia due to insulin deficiency.
  - ◇ Intercurrent illness. Unsuspected infections, including urinary tract infections and tuberculosis, may be present. Thyrotoxicosis can also manifest as unstable glycemic control.

Lactic acidosis

- The topic of lactic acidosis is beyond the scope of this book.
- It is important to know that lactic acidosis was associated with the biguanide phenformin in the past, and can occur with the use of the biguanide metformin. Though the risk of developing lactic acidosis with the use of metformin is low, the mortality rate is about 45%.
- Symptoms of lactic acidosis include anorexia, nausea, vomiting, and lethargy.
- Predisposing factors in the setting of metformin use include renal dysfunction and liver disease.
- The use of bicarbonate for treatment is controversial, and management is mainly through hemodialysis.

A combination of chaotic food intake and insulin omission is the primary cause of recurrent ketoacidosis.

CHAPTER 12

Long-term management of hyperglycemia

Overview

- Long-term management of hyperglycemia is aimed both at risk factors for complications, and at identification and treatment of complications. The broad approach includes: education, diet, exercise, oral antihyperglycemic therapy, injectables such as exenatide, and insulin.
- Patients with type 1 diabetes will generally require lifelong insulin treatment, often from the time of diagnosis.
  - ◇ Autoimmune diabetes diagnosed later in life may masquerade as type 2 and respond, at least temporarily, to oral therapy.
- In type 2 diabetes the traditional approach has been to start with diet and exercise, adding oral therapy, first as monotherapy followed by combination therapy as appropriate, with insulin being reserved until oral therapy proves insufficient, often late in the course of the disease.

- This traditional treatment paradigm could be challenged and a move made towards more aggressive and rapidly instituted early treatment. This is supported by:
  - ◇ The results of clinical trials.
  - ◇ The fact that doctors and other healthcare providers respond much too slowly to continuing inadequate glycemic control.
  - ◇ The development of new classes of drugs in the last 10 years.
- The European Association for the Study of Diabetes and the American Diabetes Association have jointly sponsored two consensus conferences on this issue, resulting in the publication of a 'treatment algorithm' for the management of hyperglycemia in type 2 diabetes (**139**).

139 Treatment algorithm. This supports the use of combination therapy and the introduction of insulin if glycemic control is not achieved. *Adapted from Nathan DM, et al, 2009.*

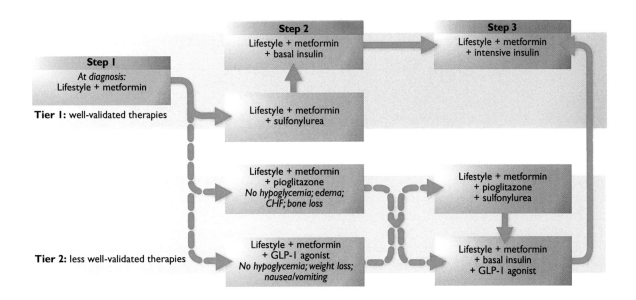

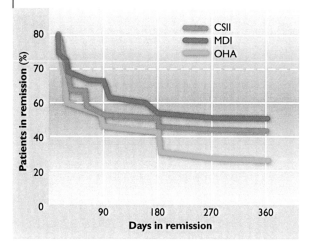

140 Intensive insulin therapy. A trial to compare the effects of continuous subcutaneous insulin infusion (CSII) or multiple daily insulin injections (MDI) with oral hypoglycemic agents (OHA) demonstrated that intensive insulin therapy in patients with newly diagnosed type 2 diabetes improves β-cell function and remission rates compared with treatment with oral hypoglycemic agents. *Adapted from Weng J et al, 2008.*

◇ This suggests that, unless there is a specific contraindication, oral antihyperglycemic therapy with metformin should be initiated, in most cases, along with lifestyle modification, as soon as diabetes has been diagnosed.

◇ The rationale for this is that lifestyle modification – essentially diet and exercise – on its own will inevitably be insufficient.

◆ This issue is bound to remain under constant scrutiny as a less didactic, more personalized approach is widely employed.

◇ For example, a recent randomized trial of temporary intensive insulin therapy versus the more traditional oral therapy at the onset of type 2 diabetes showed that both approaches will induce relatively normal blood glucose levels in the majority of patients, but the former appears to give a more sustained improvement in β-cell function and normoglycemia (**140**).

Long-term adherence to any diet plan is notoriously difficult.

Targets of treatment

◆ Targets may be set for patients to achieve weight loss, lower blood pressure and glucose levels, or improved blood lipid profile (**141, 142**).

◆ Glucose targets are usually estimated by HbA1c levels and these targets will vary with age, diabetes duration, and complication risk, including risk of hypoglycemia.

◇ The younger the patient, the lower the HbA1c; the older the patient, the higher the HbA1c (except for those under 12 years of age when recommended levels are <8.0% [64 mmol/mol] or when under 6 years of age <8.5% [69 mmol/mol]).

◇ Self-monitored blood glucose (SMBG) can improve glycemic control, particularly if it forms part of a program of patient education and staff training that promotes management adjustments according to the ensuing blood glucose values (**143**).

Dietary management

◆ The incidence of type 2 diabetes has risen in parallel with a massive increase in obesity, and it is clear that the two are causally linked.

◇ Obesity greatly increases the likelihood that a susceptible individual will develop diabetes, and failure to address the problem once diabetes has been diagnosed hampers attempts to achieve glycemic control.

◆ The main dietary issue in type 2 diabetes is that of excessive calorie intake. This problem is also becoming more prevalent in type 1 diabetes.

◆ Despite the fact that diet has long been recognized as an important issue in both type 1 and type 2 diabetes, little of the dietary advice given to patients, other than the proven benefit of calorie restriction, is truly evidence-based. It is important to observe that:

◇ Long-term adherence to any dietary plan is notoriously difficult, and this is a major stumbling block both in performing the appropriate studies and in applying the results of short-term studies.

◇ Dietary advice to patients with diabetes is largely empirical and owes much to the consensus views of 'nutritional experts' and to prevailing fashions.

Therapeutic targets

Weight	Body mass index <25 Waist:hip ratio men <0.95; women <0.8
Glucose	HbA1c <7.0% (53 mmol/mol) (but depends on age, diabetes duration, complication risk)
Lipid profile	Cholesterol <4.0 mmol/l (155 mg/dl) LDL cholesterol <2.6 mmol/l (100 mg/dl) (lower if overt vascular disease i.e. <2.0 mmol/l [70 mg/dl]) Triglycerides <1.7 mmol/l (150 mg/dl)
Blood pressure	130/80 mmHg (but depends on age, diabetes duration, complication risk)
Smoking	Nil

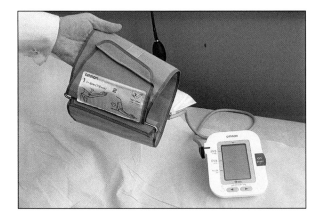

142 A large BP cuff, suitable for obese patients. Blood pressure levels are one of the clinical parameters which are used to monitor the effectiveness of diabetes management.

Plasma glucose goals for SMBG

AACE and IDF	
Fasting	<110 mg/dl (6.1 mmol/l)
2-hour postprandial	<140 mg/dl (7.8 mmol/l)
ADA and EASD	
Preprandial	70–130 mg/dl (3.9–7.2 mmol/l)
1–2 hour peak postprandial	<180 mg/dl (10 mmol/l)

AACE: American Association of Clinical Endocrinologists
ADA: American Diabetes Association
EASD: European Association for the Study of Diabetes
IDF: International Diabetes Federation

141 Therapeutic targets. These should be agreed between the patient and the healthcare team.

◆ It seems reasonable to suggest that the diet of a diabetic patient should, in principle, be no different from that considered healthy for the population as a whole, perhaps with special emphasis on the avoidance of refined sugar.
  ◇ Diet and exercise should be regarded as the cornerstone of treatment for type 2 diabetes.

Calorie intake

◆ Calorie intake should be tailored to individual patients, taking into account their weight at the time they come to medical attention.
  ◇ At diagnosis, type 1 diabetic patients will typically have lost weight and are likely to be below ideal body weight.
  ◇ Patients with type 2 diabetes will likely have had weight gain for several years, but then start losing weight in the weeks to months leading up to the diagnosis of diabetes; most remain overweight, sometimes substantially so, when diabetes is diagnosed.
  ◇ Those patients with latent autoimmune diabetes of adults (LADA), who are initially 'misdiagnosed' as having type 2 diabetes (about 8–12% of newly diagnosed adult patients), will *generally* have had more weight loss and been more symptomatic than true type 2 patients. However, the overlap between the two groups in respect of these features is considerable.
◆ A reasonable goal is to try to achieve and maintain a weight close to ideal body weight.
◆ While there are usually advantages to a 'slow and steady' approach to weight loss, others advocate using a newly diagnosed patient's high motivation to aim for more rapid loss.
◆ When considering a dietary strategy that will help achieve this it is useful to think in terms of overall calorie intake, and composition of the diet in terms of carbohydrate, protein, and fat content.

143 Self-monitored blood glucose. Glycemic goals should be individualized based on age, history, and self-management capabilities.

Long-term management of hyperglycemia

◇ An overweight patient (BMI 25–30 kg/m²) should be started on a reducing diet of approximately 4–6 J (1000–1500 kcal) daily.

◇ Opinions vary as to whether obese individuals, BMI >30 kg/m², should be advised on even greater calorie restriction; a target of 3.2–4 J (800–1000 kcal) daily is ideal, although many patients will have difficulty complying with this.

◇ In the US, where meal portions are typically greater than in most other countries, there is reluctance, among both health professionals and patients, to recommend less than 7.2 J (1800 kcal) daily.

◆ Patients who have lost weight because of untreated diabetes may require energy supplementation.

◆ Successful weight loss soon after diagnosis of type 2 diabetes was associated in one study with a reduced subsequent mortality.

Most people with type 2 diabetes will benefit from an overall reduction in calorie intake.

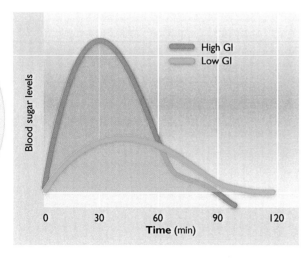

144 Glycemic index. The GI rating of a food is calculated by dividing the area under the blood glucose curve (AUC) for the test food by the AUC for the reference food (the same amount of glucose) and multiplying by 100.

Carbohydrates

◆ Diabetes diets or food plans should include unrefined carbohydrate rather than simple sugars such as sucrose.

◆ Carbohydrate is absorbed relatively slowly from fiber-rich foods, but when refined sugar is eaten the blood glucose may rise rapidly. For example, the glucose peak seen in the blood after eating an apple is much flatter than that seen after drinking the same amount of carbohydrate as apple juice (**144**).

◆ The glycemic index (GI) ranks carbohydrates according to the extent to which they raise blood sugar levels. Foods with a high GI are those which are rapidly absorbed and result in marked fluctuations in blood sugar levels. Low-GI foods, which are slow acting, produce gradual rises.

◇ Low-GI diets have been shown to improve glucose, lipid, and insulin levels in people with diabetes). They can also aid weight control by delaying hunger.

◆ An emphasis on foods with a lower GI would seem logical.

◇ For insulin-treated patients, estimating the carbohydrate content and GI of a meal may be useful in estimating the insulin requirement.

◇ This requires that patients receive education in estimating the carbohydrate content of meals, and this has now superseded the older practice of thinking in terms of 'exchanges'.

◆ The glycemic index is not universally accepted among endocrinologists, since when you take in carbohydrate, it is usually in combination with fat and protein, which often negates the value of the GI, and GI is highly dependent upon the way the food is cooked.

Fats

◆ The importance of cholesterol in the development of macrovascular disease has encouraged a more stringent attitude to fat content in diets than previously.

◇ Low-fat diets in general have only a small impact on the level of serum cholesterol, but they can be of value in limiting increases in serum triglycerides.

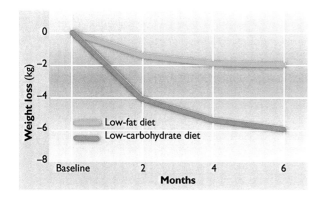

145 Low-carbohydrate vs low-fat diets. In trials comparing low-fat with low-carbohydrate diets, the latter were more effective in inducing weight loss over a 6-month period.

Prescribing a diet

◆ For most people changing the dietary habits of a lifetime is challenging, so one needs to take a sympathetic approach.
  ◇ The main point to be made to most people with type 2 diabetes is that an overall reduction in calorie intake is appropriate and will be beneficial (**146, 147**). This needs to be emphasized, even, or especially, to those patients who, despite their excess weight, insist that they do not overeat. Equivocation on the part of medical carers on this issue does a disservice to patients.

◆ Conventional wisdom has it that saturated fatty acids should be restricted to less than 10% of the total daily energy intake.
  ◇ Foods that should be restricted but not eliminated include dairy produce, chocolate, ice creams, shellfish including prawns, the fat around meat especially pork and lamb, fried foods, coconut oil, avocado, and alcohol.
◆ The whole issue of fat content of the diet has captured the public imagination over the last few years through advocacy of diet plans such as the Atkins diet or the South Beach diet. These, and other diets that have a relatively high fat content, run counter to the prevailing conventional wisdom that a diet high in carbohydrates is most appropriate for people with diabetes. Advocates of higher-fat diets would say that a greater fat content is associated with increased satiety and, therefore, improved adherence to the diet with more successful weight reduction.
  ◇ It is only quite recently that controlled studies have been performed to compare the relative merits of these different approaches; in patients with severe obesity and/or type 2 diabetes it would appear that over periods of 6–12 months relatively high-fat (low-carbohydrate) diets are at least as successful as low-fat (high-carbohydrate) diets in terms of weight loss, with no adverse effect on fasting lipid profile (**145**).
    ◇ Perhaps the most telling point in such studies is that compliance with *any* diet tends to decrease substantially beyond 6 months.

Diet recommendations

No refined sugar

Avoid 'diabetic' foods

Small frequent meals

Reduce calorie intake

Encourage complex, high-fiber carbohydrates

Limit fat intake: saturated fats <10% of total energy intake

Encourage monounsaturated fats (olive oil, rapeseed oil)

Cholesterol <250 mg/day (less if dyslipidemia)

Limit salt intake: <2.3 g per day

Limit alcohol intake: men <28 units/week; women <21 units/week

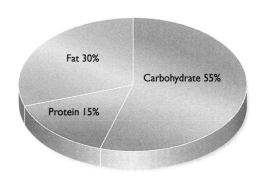

146, 147 Dietary strategies. Reduced calories and reduced fat intake can lower the risk of diabetic complications. The ratio of carbohydrate, protein, and fat can be adjusted to meet the metabolic goals and preferences of the patient.

Long-term management of hyperglycemia

- A diet history should be taken, and review of a complete 3-day diet diary, including all snacks, can lead many patients to recognize previously unappreciated sources of excess calories. Soft drinks ('sodas' in the US) and fruit juices are particularly rich 'hidden' sources of calories, particularly among younger patients.
- Another aspect of concern to many is alcohol. Alcohol should not be forbidden, but its energy content should be taken into account; aim for <28 units per week in men and <21 units per week in women.
  - In simple terms, 1 unit can be an 85 ml glass of wine, a half pint of beer, or 25 ml of spirits.
- Patients can be told that studies consistently show a significant correlation between modest alcohol intake and reduced risk of heart disease, while at the same time pointing to the hazards of excessive alcohol.
- Patients on insulin should be warned to avoid alcoholic binges since these may precipitate severe hypoglycemia, and late-evening alcohol will increase the risk of nocturnal hypoglycemia.
- A daily sodium intake of 2.3 g per day is recommended to limit the risk of hypertension.
- Foods that are labeled 'diabetic' are not recommended, as they usually contain nonglucose refined sugars such as sucrose or fructose. Artificial sweeteners are useful and could be used as an alternative to sugar; concerns that they cause cancer have not been confirmed.
- Patients on insulin or oral agents should be advised to eat the same amount at the same time each day. Patients on insulin usually require snacks between meals and at bedtime, as injected insulin may linger in the blood.

Aim for at least 30 minutes of exercise a day.

148 **Exercise guidelines.** All levels of physical activity can be undertaken by people with type 1 diabetes who do not have complications and have good glycemic control. Therapeutic regimens can be adjusted to allow safe participation consistent with an individual's goals and abilities.

Exercise

- Along with dietary change there must be an emphasis on overall lifestyle change, particularly in respect of exercise. It is useful to point out that small changes in everyday activities can be useful, for example:
  - Using stairs instead of lifts (elevators) to go up two or three floors.
  - Parking at the point furthest from one's place of work or the supermarket rather than as close as possible.
  - Doing small local errands on foot rather than always jumping into the car.
  - Getting off the bus a stop early.
  - Walking faster; walking a dog.
- Regular scheduled exercise, even if only walking, should be encouraged, perhaps even prescribed, the aim being at least a half-hour each day on average (**148**).

Exercise guidelines in type 1 diabetes

GENERAL ADVICE

Exercise regularly; even walking has metabolic benefits

Tailor exercise regime to fit individual needs and physical fitness

Avoid hypoglycemia during exercise by:
- Taking 20–40 g extra carbohydrate before and hourly during exercise
- Reduce pre-exercising insulin doses by 30–50%, if necessary
- Use nonexercising sites for injections
- Avoid heavy exercise during peak from insulin injection

CONTRAINDICATIONS

For those taking insulin, sports where hypoglycemia could be dangerous (e.g. climbing, motor racing, diving, single-handed sailing)

In those with proliferative retinopathy, strenuous exercise (due to the risk of possible hemorrhage)

CAUTIONS

Take care if cardiovascular comorbidities are present

Those with peripheral neuropathy need to be aware of the potential for damage to the feet

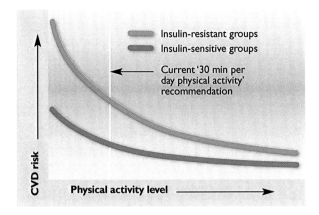

149 Physical activity and cardiovascular disease.
Dose–response relationship between physical activity level and CVD risk in normal weight nondiabetic individuals with no family history of diabetes (insulin-sensitive) and in individuals who are insulin resistant or with a predisposition to insulin resistance. Those most at risk are most likely to benefit from exercise. *Adapted from Gill JMR, Malkova D, 2006.*

◆ It is important to point out that even vigorous exercise uses up fewer calories than most people realize, and that a large soft drink or a snack can quickly cancel out the calories expended.

◆ Another point to be emphasized is that perhaps the greatest value of regular exercise, even when there is disappointingly little weight loss, is that it reduces insulin resistance and improves cardio-vascular risk (**149**, **150**). Exercise is therefore a cornerstone of diabetes therapy.

◆ When planning an exercise regime it is important to:
  ◇ Assess contraindications and limitations.
  ◇ Be realistic – people will only continue to do what they enjoy.
  ◇ Build up the amount of exercise gradually.
  ◇ Advise about the risk of hypoglycemia (**151**).
  ◇ Remember, any exercise is better than none.

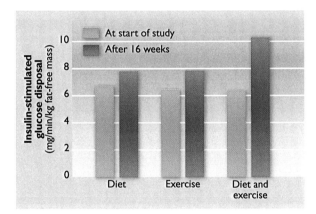

150 Exercise and insulin sensitivity. A study of 25 non-diabetic obese individuals demonstrated greater improvement in insulin sensitivity through diet and exercise combined, compared with either diet or exercise alone – possibly as a result of improved fatty acid metabolism. *Adapted from Goodpaster BH et al, 2003.*

Glycemic response to acute exercise in type 1 diabetes

BLOOD GLUCOSE LEVEL	EXERCISE CONDITIONS
Decreases	Hyperinsulinemia exists during exercise
	Exercise is intensive or prolonged (>30–60 min in duration)
	<3 h have elapsed since the preceding meal
	No extra snacks are taken before or during the exercise
Generally remains unchanged	Plasma insulin concentration is normal during exercise
	Exercise is brief
	Appropriate snacks are taken before and during exercise
Increases	Hypoinsulinemia exists during exercise
	Exercise is marked, but not prolonged
	Excessive carbohydrates are taken before and/or during exercise

Aerobic exercise improves insulin sensitivity and reduces cardiovascular risk.

151 Glycemic response. The glycemic response to exercise in people with type 1 diabetes varies between individuals and according to the intensity and duration of the exercise.

Long-term management of hyperglycemia

Bariatric surgery

- Weight loss is the cornerstone of the management of overweight and obese subjects with type 2 diabetes.
- Increasingly, patients are coming to bariatric surgery after exhausting other methods of weight control. Bariatric surgery should be considered for adults with BMI >35 kg/m², but data are insufficient to make a broad-based recommendation for surgery at lesser weights.
- There are two general types of bariatric surgery, depending on their mechanism of inducing weight loss: malabsorptive and restrictive. The following are some examples (**152**).
  - ◇ *Laparoscopic adjustable gastric banding (restrictive)*. A band is placed around the stomach, limiting its size and producing early satiety. The size of the stomach can be adjusted by injecting saline into the band.
  - ◇ *Sleeve gastrectomy (restrictive)*. The stomach is resected parallel to its greater curvature.
  - ◇ *Jejunoileal bypass (malabsorptive)*. The jejunum is divided and then connected to the ileum just proximal to the ileocecal valve.

- ◇ *Roux-en-Y gastric bypass (malabsorptive and restrictive)*. This is one of the most common procedures. A gastric pouch of around 30 ml is created and the small intestine is divided. Food drains into the distal (Roux) limb, which is connected to the gastric pouch, while the proximal limb drains secretions from the stomach remnant, liver, and pancreas. The two limbs are connected in the distal jejunum by a 'Y'-shaped anastomosis.
- Malabsorptive procedures show faster and more durable weight loss and improvement in glycemic control than restrictive procedures.
- For operations that physically limit food intake, the time course and degree of improvement in diabetes are more or less in line with predictions based on the degree of postoperative weight loss.
  - ◇ The long-term benefit of gastric banding is not substantial and the technique is being used less frequently.
- The effects of bypass procedures appear quite different. Improvements in glycemia have been reported well before weight loss becomes apparent, and in addition, exceed those expected on the basis of the amount of weight lost.
  - ◇ Increased secretion of a number of gut peptides with insulinotropic actions, such as GLP-1 and GIP, and decreased secretion of orexigenic peptides, such as ghrelin, implying gastro-endocrine effect.
- Many series purporting to show 'cure' of diabetes, often associated with restoration of first-phase insulin response in up to 80% of subjects for as long as 16 years of follow-up, have been reported. Prospective studies lacking the bias inherent in such reports are eagerly awaited.
- Patients who have had bariatric surgery need lifelong support and medical monitoring.

Long-term management of hyperglycemia

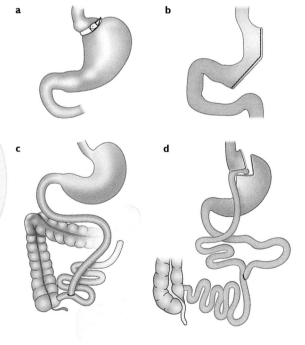

152 Types of bariatric surgery. Illustrated are the laparoscopic band (a), sleeve gastrectomy (b), jejunoileal bypass (c), and Roux-en-Y gastric bypass (d).

Bariatric surgery may be considered for adults who have exhausted other methods of weight control.

CHAPTER 13

Noninsulin therapies

Tablet treatment for type 2 diabetes

◆ Diet and lifestyle changes are the key to successful treatment of type 2 diabetes. If there can be satisfactory metabolic control by these means then tablets may not be required.

◇ The UKPDS showed, however, that an initial favorable response in most patients is transient, so that additional therapy is almost always necessary within 6 months.

◇ It can still be beneficial for many patients to undertake an initial period (up to 3–6 months) of diet and lifestyle change; this would impress on them that this is the cornerstone of treatment, and it would identify those for whom it is sufficiently successful. It is then important to guard against 'clinical inertia', with patient and medical adviser being too slow to accept the need for progressive treatment decisions.

◆ The European Association for the Study of Diabetes and the American Diabetes Association 2008 'consensus algorithm' supports oral antihyperglycemic therapy – specifically metformin – along with lifestyle modification, as the first step in treatment (see p. 131).

◇ The 2012 ADA/EASD treatment algorithm endorses the view that either a sulfonylurea, thiazolidinedione, dipeptidyl peptidase-4 (DPP-4) inhibitor, or GLP-1 analogue is appropriate 'add-on' treatment to metformin, emphasizing a personalized approach.

◇ Nevertheless, it is useful to consider the effect that a particular drug may have on β-cell function when deciding on treatment early in type 2 diabetes. Although it has not been convincingly shown that these drugs will halt or slow the decline in β-cell function in human type 2 diabetes, *in vitro* and animal studies suggest that this may be the case.

◆ There is a view that emphasis on these drugs, rather than insulin secretagogues and insulin, early in the disease course, may be more successful in preventing the long-term rise in HbA1c that was seen in the UKPDS, after the intial improvement in the first 2 years postdiagnosis, using sulfonylureas, metformin, or insulin (**153**).

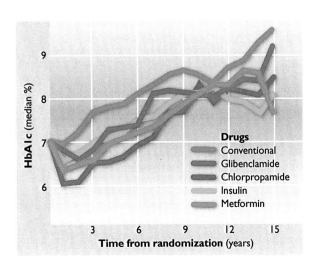

153 Effect of intensive blood-glucose control with metformin. The UKPDS group trial found that metformin appeared to decrease the risk of diabetes-related endpoints and was associated with less weight gain and fewer hypoglycemic attacks than insulin and sulfonylureas (glibenclamide and chlorpropamide). Intial responses to all agents were similar, but sulfonylureas demonstrated less later benefit.

- In practice, there can be no strict rules regarding the introduction of oral hypoglycemic agents.
  - Relief of hyperglycemia by any means will have a temporary beneficial effect on β-cell function and insulin secretion, at least early in the course of type 2 diabetes.
  - There may be differences in the degree of HbA1c lowering with the different classes, but most studies show these to be minor.
  - The HbA1c level at the start of treatment is one of the variables determining the likely magnitude of HbA1c fall; so a drug may be able to cause a reduction in HbA1c from 10% (86 mmol/mol) to 8% (64 mmol/mol), but would be unlikely to cause a reduction from 8% (64 mmol/mol) to 6% (42 mmol/mol).
- The preventive effect of any class in relation to microvascular disease almost certainly depends on the extent of improvement in glycemia.
  - To date, the UKPDS is the only study to suggest an advantage of one agent over another in terms of reducing the risk of cardiovascular disease, in that metformin-treated obese patients had fewer cardio-vascular events than those randomized to initial sulfonylurea or insulin treatment.
  - The UKPDS also confirmed that sulfonylurea monotherapy, in comparison with diet and exercise, does not increase cardiovascular risk.
  - It is unlikely that any future trials will further assess this question for monotherapy.
- The initial choice of an antidiabetic drug is often arbitrary, depending on such things as patient and physician preference, cost, and potential adverse effects. Nevertheless, the preference indicated in the EASD/ADA treatment algorithm is for metformin as the initial choice.
- Patients with baseline HbA1c >9% (75mmol/mol) are less likely to achieve target HbA1c with monotherapy and are candidates for the early introduction of combination therapy, even going straight from diet and exercise to combination therapy.
- The natural history of type 2 diabetes suggests that insulin secretory capacity is already decreased by 50% or more on average at the time of diagnosis and it can be expected to continue decreasing for at least 6 years after that (**154**).
- Since type 2 diabetes is characterized by both diminished insulin secretion and increased insulin resistance it makes sense to target each of these defects at an early stage, and the most common combination currently prescribed is metformin plus a sulfonylurea. However, this traditional paradigm could well change.
- Inhaled insulin did not prove an attractive option to many patients as an alternative to stimulating endogenous insulin secretion, and the market leader, Exubera, was withdrawn in the US for commercial reasons.
- These points serve to illustrate how the rapidly evolving therapeutic options are 'complicating' treatment paradigms that came into practice more due to what was available than to what was necessarily best for the patient.
- The challenge facing patients and their medical advisers is to keep pace with their changing needs by whatever combinations of therapy prove effective and to avoid the clinical inertia mentioned above. An understanding of the merits and potential adverse effects of each of the various classes of drugs is therefore essential (**155**).

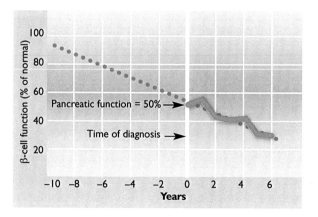

154 Decline in β-cell function. The UKPDS showed that newly diagnosed people with type 2 diabetes had, on average, only about 50% of normal β-cell insulin-secretory function, with a further progressive fall in the years of follow-up. By extrapolating backward (dotted line), it was estimated that this β-cell defect had begun 5–10 years before diagnosis.

Non-insulin diabetes medications

DRUG	BENEFITS	RISKS
Oral therapies Metformin	Weight gain not common; might result in weight loss; low risk of hypoglycemia when used alone; inexpensive; may reduce HbA1c by 1.5–2%	Contraindicated in renal dysfunction, acute heart failure, or other conditions that predispose to lactic acidosis; gastrointestinal side effects are common
Insulin secretagogues: sulfonylureas	Inexpensive; may reduce HbA1c by 1.5–2%	Hypoglycemia is common; may cause weight gain
Insulin secretagogues: nateglinide, repaglinide	Weight gain seems to be less than with sulfonylureas	Hypoglycemia may occur
Thiazolidinedione	Reduces insulin resistance; low risk of hypoglycemia when used alone	May cause weight gain and fluid retention; mild anemia; increased risk of limb fracture and microfracture; contraindicated in heart failure and in patients with bladder cancer
Alpha-glucosidase inhibitors	Weight gain not common	Gastrointestinal side-effects are common
DPP-4 inhibitors	Low risk of hypoglycemia when given alone or with metformin or thiazolidinediones; weight gain not common	Rare cases of angioedema and Stevens–Johnson syndrome have been reported
Colesevelam	Lowers cholesterol and glucose levels (though HbA1c reduction only 0.5–0.6% on average)	Gastrointestinal side-effects are common
Bromocriptine	Low risk of hypoglycemia	Nausea and dizziness are common
Injectables GLP-1 analogs: exenatide, liraglutide	Weight loss is common	Nausea is common at first; possible association with pancreatitis; liraglutide contraindicated if there is a history of medullary thyroid carcinoma and in patients with multiple endocrine neoplasia 2
Pramlintide	Might result in weight loss	Nausea is common at first; contraindicated in confirmed gastroparesis and hypoglycemia unawareness

Metformin

155 Anti-diabetic drug choices. The benefits and risks of the types of glucose-lowering agents are summarized.

◆ Metformin is a biguanide. Its mechanism of action is unclear, but it decreases gluconeogenesis and hence hepatic glucose output and fasting blood glucose. It increases glucose uptake in skeletal muscle. These effects are mediated, at least in part, by AMPK activation.

◆ Metformin has been in use in most countries for about 40 years, but gained FDA approval in the US only in 1995.

◆ Metformin is the drug of preference in overweight type 2 diabetic subjects:

◇ The UKPDS led to renewed enthusiasm for metformin, as it was associated with reduced cardiovascular risk in overweight patients, especially as monotherapy.

◇ Metformin is associated with less weight gain than other agents, with some patients actually losing weight while glycemic control improves.

Noninsulin therapies

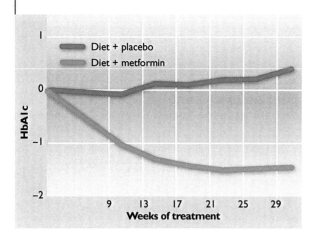

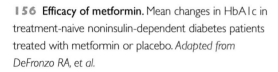

156 Efficacy of metformin. Mean changes in HbA1c in treatment-naive noninsulin-dependent diabetes patients treated with metformin or placebo. *Adapted from DeFronzo RA, et al.*

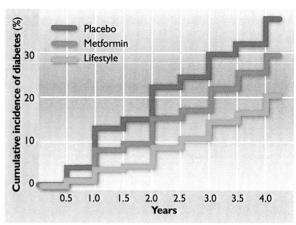

157 Metformin vs lifestyle intervention. In the DPP study, the cumulative incidence of diabetes was lower in the metformin and lifestyle-intervention groups than in the placebo group throughout the follow-up period. *Adapted from Knowler WC et al.*

◆ As monotherapy it typically reduces HbA1c by 1.5–2% depending on baseline level, and in patients with type 2 diabetes on insulin treatment it reduces HbA1c by about 1% (**156**).

◆ Metformin can be used in combination with all other diabetic drugs.
  ◇ Even obese patients with type 1 diabetes may benefit in terms of reduced HbA1c from using metformin.

◆ Its dose–response relationship is linear up to a dose of 2000 mg per day, usually given as 1000 mg morning and evening.
  ◇ In Europe (but not in America) doses up to 3000 mg per day are sometimes prescribed; at levels above 2000 mg per day there is little further hypoglycemic effect, though there may be an effect on lipids, particularly triglycerides.

◆ The ability of metformin to prevent or delay the onset of diabetes in subjects at increased risk (with impaired glucose tolerance) was suggested in the Diabetes Prevention Program, in which over 3000 subjects with pre-diabetes – defined as elevated fasting and post-glucose-load plasma glucose – were randomly assigned to lifestyle intervention, metformin, or placebo (no intervention), and the incidence of diabetes was observed over 4 years (**157**).

◇ The drug did reduce the risk of diabetes being diagnosed by 31% over a 4-year period when compared with placebo, but was not as effective as a supervised program of lifestyle change (diet and exercise), which reduced the likelihood of diabetes by 58% compared with placebo.

◇ As yet, the prescription of metformin in this situation is not generally approved or agreed.

Side-effects

◆ The major side-effects are abdominal discomfort, nausea, and diarrhea.
  ◇ These problems are idiosyncratic and often dose-related; they can be limited by initiating therapy at a low dose (500 mg daily), taking the drug with food, and then titrating gradually to the maximally tolerated dose, or by using a modified-release formulation.

◆ Because its mode of action does not involve increased insulin secretion, hypoglycemia is rarely a problem when metformin is used as monotherapy. In combination with insulin or insulin secretagogues the risk is greater, and in those circumstances it makes sense to adjust the dosage of the other drug rather than to give metformin at less than optimal levels.

- A rare complication of biguanide therapy is the development of lactic acidosis, which can be fatal. This was seen more commonly with phenformin, another biguanide with metabolic effects significantly different from those of metformin. The risk of precipitating lactic acidosis is extremely low in otherwise healthy individuals.
  - ◇ Metformin is contraindicated in renal or hepatic disease or where there is increased risk of lactic acidosis. Guidelines caution against its use in patients with a serum creatinine >130 µmol/l (1.5 mg/dl).
  - ◇ The FDA has been monitoring carefully for an increase in the reported cases of lactic acidosis in the US, and, to date, none has been recorded, even though significant numbers of patients with elevated serum creatinine receive the drug; similar data are available from Scotland.
  - ◇ Particular care should be taken in the elderly and in those with decreased muscle mass because serum creatinine tends to underestimate the degree of renal impairment in such patients.
- Metformin should be discontinued the day before and for 24 hours after radiological contrast use or surgical procedures. It should also be interrupted in severe illnesses.

Insulin secretagogues: sulfonylureas

- Sulfonylureas increase insulin secretion from the pancreatic β cell by closing ATP-sensitive potassium (K_{ATP}) channels, depolarizing the β-cell plasma membrane, and increasing intracellular calcium concentration (**158**).
  - ◇ Other insulin secretagogues have essentially the same mechanism of action.
- Sulfonylureas are effective in decreasing both fasting blood glucose and postprandial hyperglycemia.
- About 20% of patients have little or no glycemic response to sulfonylureas.
- It has been said that some patients (perhaps 30%) eventually cease to respond to these drugs, leading to the concept of 'sulfonylurea failure'. Evidence for this is marginal at best, and studies in patients treated long term who then discontinue treatment invariably show a rise in HbA1c, indicating that the drug was still having an effect.
  - ◇ The term 'sulfonylurea failure' really relates to failure of the drug, either on its own or in combination with another agent, to achieve the desired degree of glycemic control; this is not a reason to discontinue the drug.

Stop metformin 24 hours before and after radiological contrast use or surgical procedures.

158 Sulfonylurea action. Sulfonylureas inhibit the outflow of potassium from the K_{ATP} channels, leading to the depolarization of the cell membrane, the opening of the Ca^{2+} channels, and an increased secretion of insulin.

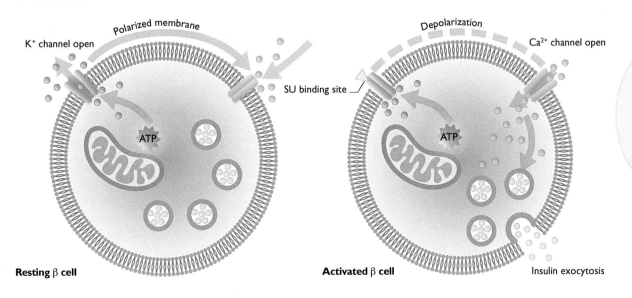

K⁺ channel open — Polarized membrane

SU binding site

ATP

Resting β cell

Depolarization — Ca²⁺ channel open

ATP

Activated β cell

Insulin exocytosis

Noninsulin therapies

- Until the resurgent popularity of metformin, sulfonylureas had been the first choice for oral monotherapy. Just as with metformin, sulfonylureas typically cause HbA1c levels to drop by 1.5–2% as monotherapy, with smaller decreases when added to other agents.
- With all sulfonylureas most of the hypoglycemic effect is achieved at low doses; addition of a drug from another class will usually produce a greater fall in HbA1c than increasing the dose of sulfonylurea from minimum starting dose to the maximum approved.
- Because sulfonylureas stimulate insulin release it is tempting to think that they would be most appropriate when insulin deficiency is the predominant factor, and that they would be less effective in patients with insulin resistance.
  - ◇ Measurement of the extent of these dual impairments is imprecise even under controlled research conditions, and is simply beyond the scope of day-to-day practice; since both are present to some degree in most type 2 diabetes patients, a sulfonylurea almost always represents a reasonable treatment option.
- One rare indication for sulfonylureas is for patients with neonatal diabetes due to potassium channel gene mutations; in these children, sulfonylureas can circumvent the defect in stimulus–secretion coupling, so that insulin secretion can be restored and insulin therapy stopped.
- Several sulfonylurea drugs are available for prescription.
  - ◇ Chlorpropamide has a biological half-life measured in days, and is rarely prescribed now.
  - ◇ Glibenclamide (glyburide in the US), glipizide, glimepiride, and gliclazide all have the advantage of being effective on a once-daily dosage though they are often prescribed in split doses when using the maximum dosage.

Drug interactions and side-effects

- Sulfonylureas bind to circulating albumin, and they may be displaced by other drugs that compete for their binding sites, e.g. warfarin.
- Hypoglycemia, particularly during the late postprandial period or at night, is the most common and dangerous side-effect and, despite the relatively poor dose–response relationship mentioned above, tends to be dose-dependent.
  - ◇ Because the effect of many sulfonylureas persists for more than 24 hours, chlorpropamide in particular, recurrent or prolonged hypoglycemia is likely, and hospital admission may be advisable.
  - ◇ Impaired renal and hepatic function increase the risk of hypoglycemia, especially with chlorpropamide and glibenclamide, so sulfonylureas should be used with care in patients with renal and liver disease. Gliclazide is the preferred sulfonylurea in patients with impaired renal function, and glyburide should definitely be avoided.
  - ◇ The elderly are also at greater risk of hypoglycemia, probably due to decreased renal function and slower clearance of most sulfonylureas; glibenclamide, in particular, has been associated with severe hypoglycemia in the elderly with impaired renal function.
- Many patients will gain weight with sulfonylurea treatment.
  - ◇ In large part this is due to decreased urine glucose wasting as blood glucose levels fall to below the renal threshold for glycosuria.
  - ◇ It may also occur because subclinical hypoglycemia, which can occur with all sulfonylureas, may stimulate appetite.
- Rash can occur, though it is not common, and it is dose-independent.
- Patients who have had allergy to sulfonamides should avoid sulfonylureas.

Hypoglycemia is the most common and dangerous side-effect of sulfonylureas.

Sulfonylureas and heart disease

◆ Concern that sulfonylurea treatment may increase the risk of heart disease in type 2 diabetes, raised by the University Group Diabetes Program (UGDP) in the 1960s, has waned.
  ◇ The UKPDS found no increase in reported cardiovascular deaths in patients randomized to monotherapy with sulfonylurea.
  ◇ Treating nondiabetic dogs with sulfonylurea has been shown to reduce or abolish 'ischemic preconditioning', the process whereby repeated episodes of ischemia before occlusion of the coronary artery lead to a smaller infarct size than if there has been no previous ischemia.
  ◇ Retrospective studies in patients with diabetes have shown a worse prognosis following acute coronary syndrome in those treated with sulfonylurea before the event, but there are insufficient prospective data.
◆ Sulfonylureas differ in their affinity for the K_{ATP} channels on heart muscle cells; there is some support for the use of a sulfonylurea with a low affinity for heart receptors, such as glimepiride.
◆ A general consensus is that any type 2 diabetic patient admitted to hospital with an acute myocardial infarction should have insulin treatment aimed at achieving near-normal glycemia in place of sulfonylurea treatment.

159 Chemical structure of repaglinide and nateglinide. Both these agents have a benzamido group which binds to the sulfonylurea receptor on the β-cell membrane.

Nateglinide

Repaglinide

◆ Two drugs in this category are currently available, repaglinide and nateglinide (**159**). They belong to two similar, though not identical, classes of drugs, but are often grouped together as meglitinides or 'glinides'.
◆ These drugs can be used as initial monotherapy or in combination with other oral agents such as metformin or TZDs (see below).
◆ They work by closing the K_{ATP} channels on the β-cell membrane and stimulating glucose-dependent insulin secretion, which is quickly reversed when glucose levels fall.
  ◇ This action is more rapid in onset than that of the sulfonylureas, significantly decreasing postprandial hyperglycemia when taken shortly before each meal.
  ◇ However, because of their relatively short duration of action, these drugs have less effect on fasting glucose. This may explain why, despite their effect on postprandial insulin secretion, they have no greater ability to lower HbA1c than do the sulfonylureas. In fact, in a head-to-head trial, nateglinide as monotherapy lowered HbA1c less than glibenclamide.
◆ The effects of these drugs on vascular mortality in diabetes is unknown, although there is no reason to think they would be detrimental.

Side-effects

◆ Weight gain may be less than with sulfonylureas although full comparative studies are not yet available.
◆ As with any drug that stimulates the K_{ATP} channels, hypoglycemia is possible. It was initially hoped that their rapid onset and shorter duration of action would eliminate the risk of nocturnal hypoglycemia, but this can occur, at least with repaglinide.
◆ There is evidence that patients with the most common form of MODY (HNF-1α mutations) (see p. 18) suffer less from hypoglycemia on these agents than they do with sulfonylureas, and therefore they may be the treatment of choice for this condition.

Noninsulin therapies

Thiazolidinediones

- The thiazolidinediones (more conveniently known as 'glitazones' or TZDs) act on the peroxisome proliferator-activated receptors (PPARs), particularly PPAR-γ. These nuclear receptors regulate DNA expression including genes involved in lipid metabolism (**160**).
- Two different heterozygous mutations that damage the function of PPAR-γ have been identified in patients with severe insulin resistance, type 2 diabetes, and hypertension at an unusually early age. These loss-of-function mutations provide genetic evidence that this receptor is important in the control of insulin sensitivity and blood pressure.
- The precise mechanism by which TZDs increase insulin sensitivity in the peripheral tissues is unclear.
  - ◇ It is known that they promote the development of mature adipocytes.
  - ◇ Subcutaneous fat is increased in comparison to visceral adiposity, although whether glitazones actually decrease visceral fat mass is less clear.
  - ◇ Concomitant with these changes there is a rise in serum adiponectin levels, which are usually decreased in type 2 diabetes and insulin resistance compared with the levels seen in nondiabetic subjects and the nonobese.

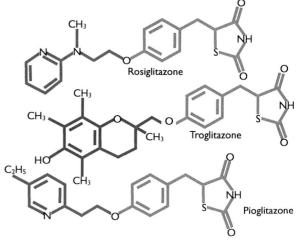

161 Chemical structure of TZDs. All the members of this class of drugs are derived from the parent compound thiazolidinedione.

- TZDs (**161**) were introduced in the late 1990s, but troglitazone was withdrawn in the UK in 1997 and the USA in 2000, due to adverse liver effects. Rosiglitazone was withdrawn in the UK in 2010 over concerns about its cardiovascular safety; in 2011 it was removed from the market in New Zealand and its use in the USA has been severely restricted. Pioglitazone is still available.
- TZDs improve glycemic control in patients with insulin resistance when used either as monotherapy or in combination with other antidiabetic agents in type 2 diabetes.
- As monotherapy their glucose-lowering effect is similar to that of other oral agents. In type 2 diabetes the addition of a glitazone to insulin treatment can further reduce the HbA1c by about 1%; in this situation particular care should be exercised because of fluid retention (see below) and in the UK this combination is not licensed.

160 PPARs. These are a group of receptor proteins found in the cell nucleus; three types (α, γ, and δ) have been identified. PPAR-γ is linked to type 2 diabetes.

Peroxisome proliferator-activated receptors (PPARs)

	PPAR-α	PPAR-δ	PPAR-γ
Tissue expression profile	Liver, kidney, skeletal muscle, brown adipose tissue	Ubiquitous	Adipose tissues, skeletal muscle, heart, liver, kidney, gut, macrophages, vascular smooth muscle cells (VSMCs)
Isoforms	α	δ	γ1, γ2
Pharmacologic activators	Fibrates, hypolipidemics		Thiazolidinediones

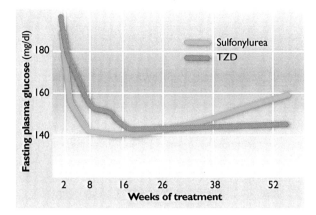

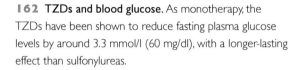

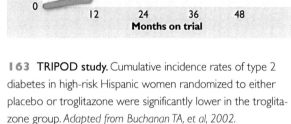

162 TZDs and blood glucose. As monotherapy, the TZDs have been shown to reduce fasting plasma glucose levels by around 3.3 mmol/l (60 mg/dl), with a longer-lasting effect than sulfonylureas.

163 TRIPOD study. Cumulative incidence rates of type 2 diabetes in high-risk Hispanic women randomized to either placebo or troglitazone were significantly lower in the troglitazone group. *Adapted from Buchanan TA, et al, 2002.*

◆ TZDs have a slower onset of action than other antihyperglycemic agents, taking several weeks to achieve their full effect, but it is possible the effect may be more durable than is the case with other oral agents (**162**).

◆ TZDs have a synergistic effect with metformin, showing that they act by a different mechanism.

◆ As with metformin, there has been speculation that, because of their mode of action, TZDs might prevent or delay the onset of diabetes.

  ◇ The TRIPOD (Troglitazone in the Prevention of Diabetes) study recruited Hispanic women who had had gestational diabetes, but who subsequently were shown not to be diabetic after the index pregnancy; compared with placebo, troglitazone led to a 58% reduction in the incidence of diabetes over a 2.4-year mean treatment period (**163**).

  ◇ A similar protective effect against the development of type 2 diabetes has been observed for pioglitazone.

◆ Patients with more insulin resistance may be expected to get the greatest benefit.

  ◇ The precise assessment of insulin resistance (and insulin secretion) is not done in routine clinical practice, but simple observations such as degree of obesity (particularly central), dyslipidemia, and acanthosis nigricans can serve as surrogate markers of increased insulin resistance.

Side-effects

◆ TZDs often cause weight gain, due to a combination of increased adipose tissue and fluid retention. Co-prescription with metformin may limit the weight gain, but it is a significant problem for many, who are already overweight to begin with.

  ◇ The increased adiposity is distributed mainly subcutaneously, and particularly at the limb girdles.

  ◇ Fluid retention may be seen, and the precise cause of this is uncertain, but it can be severe enough to precipitate heart failure, as confirmed by the PROactive study (see below), particularly in patients already on insulin treatment.

◆ Mild anemia may also occur, and it is hypothesized that this is at least partly due to hemodilution associated with fluid retention.

◆ Studies have shown an increased risk of limb fracture in women treated with TZDs, as a result of bone loss.

  ◇ The precise pathophysiology is uncertain, but it may relate to the TZDs leading precursor cells to develop preferentially into adipocytes rather than osteocytes.

◆ Recent data suggest that pioglitazone is associated with an increased risk of bladder cancer, and hence is contraindicated in at-risk patients. The etiology is not yet clear.

Noninsulin therapies

TZDs and cardiovascular disease

◆ A completed study of pioglitazone compared with placebo showed that it reduced cardiovascular events in patients with type 2 diabetes who already had documented vascular disease (the PROactive study). There was no significant difference in outcome so far as the primary endpoint was concerned, though pioglitazone treatment was associated with a significant decrease in a composite of cardiovascular death, stroke, and nonfatal myocardial infarction. This was offset, however, by an increase in the incidence of, and hospitalization for, heart failure.

◆ Set against these observations has been a controversial meta-analysis suggesting that rosiglitazone can increase not only the risk of heart failure but also of cardiovascular mortality.

◆ At the time of writing, the issue of whether TZDs will increase or reduce vascular disease remains a controversial one.

◆ Acarbose and miglitol are the two currently available drugs in this class.

◆ Alpha-glucosidase inhibitors can reduce postprandial hyperglycemia by inhibiting breakdown and digestion of complex carbohydrates in the small bowel (**164**). Because of their mode of action they are generally ineffective in patients eating either very high or very low amounts of monosaccharides.

◆ The reduction in HbA1c levels is modest compared with other oral agents, limiting their use.

◆ These drugs may have potential to reduce the risk of diabetes.
   ◇ In the STOP-NIDDM trial, treatment of people with IGT with the drug acarbose reduced the risk of developing diabetes by 25% over 3 years (**165**).

Side-effects

◆ Side-effects also tend to restrict their clinical usefulness.

◆ Undigested starch enters the large intestine, where it is broken down by fermentation causing abdominal discomfort, flatulence, and diarrhea.
   ◇ Dosage needs careful adjustment to avoid these side-effects.

◆ As little or no acarbose enters the circulation – it is mainly inactivated in the gut – other side-effects are rare, but liver dysfunction may occasionally occur with high doses.

Alpha-glucosidase inhibitors are of potential value in limiting progression to diabetes.

Intestinal villus
Acarbose
Sucrose
Fructose
Glucose
α-glucosidase
Mivcrovilli
Enterocyte

Noninsulin therapies

164 **Action of alpha-glucosidase inhibitors.** Acarbose competitively inhibits alpha-glucosidases, enzymes found in the brush border (microvilli) of the enterocytes that break down complex carbohydrates into simpler sugars. This leads to delayed absorption of carbohydrates in the intestine.

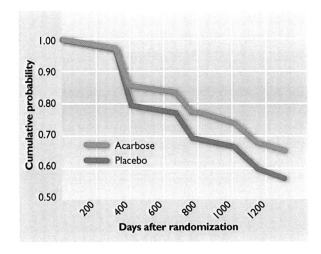

165 Alpha-glucosidase inhibitors. Patients with impaired glucose tolerance assigned to acarbose in the STOP-NIDDM randomized trial were 25% less likely to develop diabetes than those on placebo. This effect was noted at 1 year and continued throught the study. *Adapted from Chiasson et al, 2002.*

GLP-1 analogs

◆ Incretins – notably GIP and GLP-1, secreted respectively from the K and L cells of the small and large intestines – are gut hormones that enhance insulin secretion in a glucose-dependent fashion in response to ingested food (**166**).

◆ GIP and GLP-1 are rapidly (within minutes) inactivated *in vivo* by the enzyme DPP-4.

◆ Up to approximately 60% of postprandial insulin secretion is due to the incretin effect (**167**). This accounts for the long-established observation that insulin secretion is greater after ingestion of an oral glucose load than after intravenous injection of an equivalent glucose load.

◇ This effect is present, but diminished, in patients with type 2 diabetes.

166 The enteroinsular axis. Metabolic, neural, and hormonal signals are transmitted postprandially from the small intestine to the endocrine pancreas. These gut hormones – incretins – stimulate the production of insulin and inhibit that of glucagon.

Up to 60% of postprandial insulin secretion is due to the incretin effect.

---

167 The incretin effect. Orally administered glucose has a greater effect on insulin secretion than when it is given intravenously owing to the action of glucose on gut hormones. This augmented insulin secretion – the incretin effect – comprises up to 60% of postprandial insulin secretion and is diminished in type 2 diabetes.

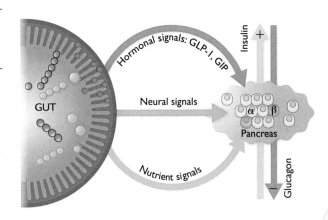

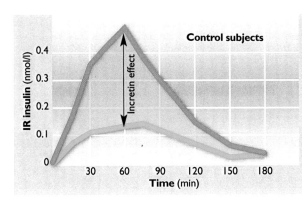

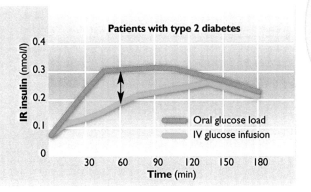

Noninsulin therapies

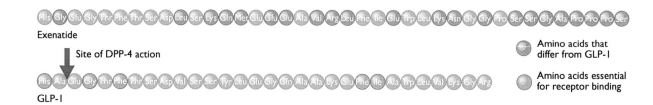

Exenatide

Site of DPP-4 action

GLP-1

○ Amino acids that differ from GLP-1

○ Amino acids essential for receptor binding

168 GLP-1 analogs. Exenatide is a 39-amino acid peptide, having 50% homology with human GLP-1. Comparative amino acid sequences of exenatide and GLP-1, and the cleavage site of DPP-4 (arrow) are shown.

GLP-1 analogs enhance insulin secretion and help reduce postprandial hyperglycemia.

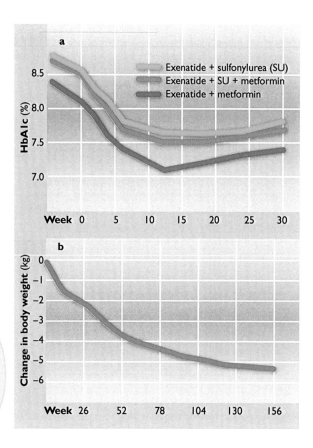

169 Exenatide. In clinical trials, exenatide was effective in lowering HbA1c by approximately 1%, when administered with sulfonylurea and/or metformin (a). Over a 3-year period it was also shown to reduce body weight by around 5 kg (b).

◆ GLP-1 is the best characterized of the incretins, and in addition to enhancing insulin secretion it suppresses production of the counter-regulatory hormone glucagon, delays gastric emptying, and induces a feeling of greater satiety. The net effect of these actions is to help limit the extent and duration of postprandial hyperglycemia.

◆ GLP-1 secretion is decreased in type 2 diabetes, making it potentially a target for therapeutic intervention.

◆ Exenatide is a synthetic form of exendin-4, a circulating meal-related peptide isolated originally from the saliva of *Heloderma suspectum* (the Gila monster). It shares slightly more than 50% homology with human GLP-1 and binds to and stimulates human GLP-1 receptors *in vitro*. Because of the difference at the site of DPP-4 action, exenatide is not inactivated by the enzyme, and therefore has a much longer half-life than native GLP-1 (**168**).

◇ Bydureon, a long-acting form of exenatide, can be given once weekly and has fewer initial side-effects.

◆ Liraglutide is an acylated form of GLP-1 given once daily with comparable glucose-lowering effects to exenatide, probably with less nausea.

◆ Subcutaneous injection of exenatide before meals is associated with enhanced insulin secretion, diminished glucagon secretion, and a decreased postprandial glucose excursion in patients with type 2 diabetes.

◇ Clinical trials of exenatide in patients with type 2 diabetes already treated with metformin, sulfonylurea, or a combination of the two, achieved a mean drop in HbA1c of approximately 1%, dependent on the initial HbA1c, for example, from 8.5% (69 mmol/mol) to 7.5% (58 mmol/mol) (**169**).

◇ Short-term studies also confirm that exenatide is effective in combination with a TZD, as is liraglutide.

Noninsulin therapies

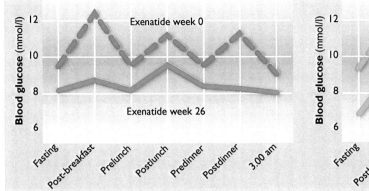

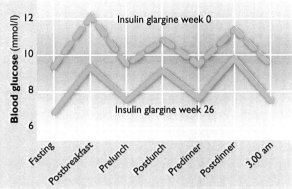

170 Exenatide and glucose levels. In this study, patients treated with exenatide had greater reduction in postprandial glucose than those treated with insulin glargine, but higher fasting glucose.

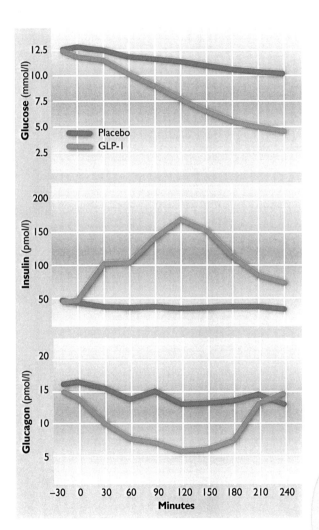

◆ Concomitant with this there is decreased appetite, and significant weight loss occurs in approximately 85% of patients treated. For those who remain on exenatide the weight loss may continue, at least up to 3 years – longer-term data are not yet available.

◆ Injection of exenatide also reduces an elevated fasting glucose.

◇ A randomized study comparing the addition of exenatide with that of insulin glargine in patients treated with oral hypoglycemic agents showed convincingly that exenatide has a much greater effect on postprandial glucose while insulin glargine has a significantly greater effect on fasting glucose (**170**).

◇ The combination of a GLP-I analog with basal insulin, together with oral agents, appears a logical and effective option, and in 2011 the FDA approved this indication for exenatide.

◆ Several other GLP-1 mimetics and analogs are under development at this time.

Side-effects

◆ An advantage of exenatide is that its effect on insulin secretion is glucose-dependent; as blood glucose falls so the effect declines, thereby reducing the risk of hypoglycemia as a side-effect (**171**).

171 Exenatide and normalization of fasting hyperglycemia. The effects of GLP-1 on insulin and glucagon secretion are glucose-dependent. An infusion of GLP-1 causes an immediate rise in insulin and a decrease in glucagon, with a resulting decrease in glucose. As glucose levels approach normal values, the insulin decreases and the glucagon increases.

Noninsulin therapies

◇ Nevertheless, when given in combination with oral agents, particularly sulfonylureas, hypoglycemia may occur, necessitating reduction in the dose of the oral agent.

◆ The major adverse effects of GLP-I analogs are nausea and vomiting, affecting 44% and 13% of subjects respectively in clinical trials of exenatide. These side effects are usually relatively short-lived, settling within 2–4 weeks, but clinical experience shows that at least 10% of patients are unwilling to persist with the drug because of them.

   ◇ A longer-acting form of the medication (Bydureon) is reported to be better tolerated.
   ◇ Side-effects of nausea and vomiting are less prevalent with liraglutide, and decline sharply in frequency if tolerated for 2 weeks.

◆ Other side-effects include diarrhea, headache, feeling jittery, and dyspepsia.

◆ In 2006 the FDA received reports of acute pancreatitis occurring in patients receiving exenatide treatment. In approximately 90% of these reports there appeared to be another well-recognized pancreatitis risk factor, such as gallstones, heavy alcohol intake, or hypertriglyceridemia.

   ◇ Whilst it seems prudent to regard pancreatitis as a potential, though uncommon, serious side-effect of these agents, there is a significant risk of pancreatitis in obese diabetes patients irrespective of therapy.

◆ Liraglutide causes thyroid C-cell tumors in rodents. However, thyroid C-cells in humans show much lower expression of GLP-1 receptors than in rodents and, to date, there has been no evidence of an increased incidence of medullary thyroid carcinoma in patients treated with liraglutide; even so, continued vigilance is advised.

DPP-4 inhibitors prolong and optimize the physiological action of GLP-1.

Dipeptidyl peptidase-4 inhibitors

◆ As mentioned above, GLP-1 is rapidly degraded by the enzyme dipeptidyl peptidase-4 (DPP-4), giving it a half-life of less than 2 minutes, so an alternative therapeutic approach is to block the action of DPP-4, thus prolonging and optimizing the physiological action of GLP-1 (**172**).

◆ Glitins approved for therapeutic use include sitagliptin, vildagliptin, saxagliptin and linagliptin.

◆ Given orally, a single dose will suppress DPP-4 activity by more than 80% for 24 hours.

   ◇ The recommended dose is 100 mg daily.

◆ In patients with type 2 diabetes, gliptins – either as monotherapy or as add-on therapy to metformin or TZD – will reduce HbA1c by, on average, 0.6–1.0% over a 3–6-month period.

◆ When given as monotherapy at full dose gliptins are almost as effective as metformin monotherapy at a dose of 500 mg twice a day, but have a lesser effect on HbA1c than metformin at 1000 mg twice a day.

◆ When the two drugs are used in combination at maximal doses as initial oral therapy, HbA1c will often be lowered by more than 2% (**173**).

◆ As might be predicted, there is a greater effect on postprandial than on fasting glucose.

◆ Gliptins in combination with sulfonylureas will reduce HbA1c, but less effectively than in combination with metformin.

   ◇ Patients with mild renal dysfunction could consider saxagliptin or linagliptin as they are not excreted by the kidneys.
   ◇ In cases of severe renal failure consider linagliptin (which is the only oral drug currently licensed for this use).

◆ Preliminary data from *in vitro* and animal studies suggest that the incretins may have a physiological role in β-cell proliferation and apoptosis. That incretin mimetics or DPP-4 inhibitors may help sustain β-cell mass in diabetic patients is therapeutically exciting, but further human studies are required to substantiate this idea.

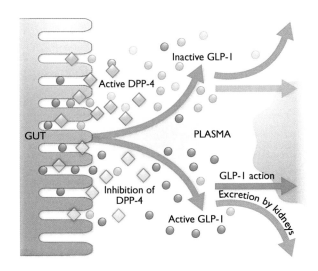

172 Action of DPP-4 inhibitors. The DPP-4 enzyme rapidly inactivates and degrades GLP-1. Gliptins bind to DPP-4, allowing the GLP-1 to remain active for longer and enhancing the endogenous incretin effect.

173 Effectiveness of DPP-4 inhibitors. This 24-week study found that a combination of sitagliptin (S) with metformin (M) therapy significantly improved glycemic control in type 2 diabetes patients. *Adapted from Goldstein BJ, et al.*

Side-effects

◆ Sitagliptin was well tolerated by patients in the pivotal clinical trials leading to its approval for general prescription. When given as monotherapy or as add-on treatment with metformin or TZD the incidence of all recorded adverse events, including hypoglycemia, was not significantly different from that seen with placebo. The absence of an increased occurrence of hypoglycemia with monotherapy no doubt reflects the glucose-dependent nature of incretin activity.

  ◇ Hypoglycemia may occur with concomitant sulfonylurea treatment.

◆ In contrast to the incretin mimetic, exenatide, gliptins do not seem to cause significant gastrointestinal side-effects.

  ◇ The difference is likely due to the fact that gliptins enhance the physiological incretin effect, whereas exenatide results in a pharmacological supranormal GLP-1-like action. This probably explains also why gliptins lack the weight-reducing effect of exenatide.

◆ Postmarketing surveillance suggests that mild headache may be the commonest side-effect.

◆ Of potentially greater importance, there have been several reports of hypersensitivity reactions including angioedema and Stevens–Johnson syndrome; the frequency seems rare, though precise figures are not available.

Other recent developments

Colesevelam

◆ Colesevelam hydrochloride, the bile acid sequestrant used to treat hyperlipidemia, was approved in 2008 in the US (but not as yet in Europe) for the treatment of type 2 diabetes in conjunction with insulin or other oral agents.

◆ The average improvement in HbA1c is 0.5–0.6%, though a reduction of 1% has been seen in those with baseline HbA1c >8% (64 mmol/mol).

◆ The speculated mechanisms include a reduction in gastrointestinal glucose absorption and effects on the incretins.

Side-effects

◆ Gastrointestinal side-effects, such as constipation and dyspepsia, are common.

◆ Its use is contraindicated in patients with a history of bowel obstruction, severe hypertriglyceridemia (>5.65 mmol/l [500 mg/dl]), and hypertriglyceridemia-induced acute pancreatitis.

Noninsulin therapies

Bromocriptine

- The quick-release form of bromocriptine (Cycloset®), a dopamine-D2-receptor agonist, has been approved by the FDA for the management of type 2 diabetes. Though the exact mechanism of its glucose-lowering effect is not known, several observations are noteworthy:
  - ◇ In patients with type 2 diabetes, it is believed that there is a decrease in dopaminergic activity, and an increase in sympathetic activity (with concomitant increase in hepatic glucose output), in the early morning.
  - ◇ In obese individuals, there is also an increase in daytime plasma prolactin levels.
  - ◇ With the administration of Cycloset in the morning, the elevated prolactin levels are reduced, possibly reflecting a restoration of dopaminergic tone, and a reduction in post-prandial plasma glucose levels.
- Bromocriptine is taken in the morning within two hours of awakening, with food. The initial dose is 0.8 mg per day and can be increased weekly, to a maximum dose of 4.8 mg per day.

Side-effects

- Bromocriptine may cause hypotension, may exacerbate psychotic disorders, and may increase the risk of hypotension in patients with syncopal migraine. There is early evidence that cardiovascular events might be decreased in patients taking Cycloset compared to placebo.

Pramlintide

- Amylin is a hormone that is co-secreted with insulin by the pancreatic β cells (see chapter 4); it has been found to reduce glucagon levels after meals, increase satiety, and delay gastric emptying. It is reduced in patients with type 2 diabetes.
- Pramlintide, an amylin analog, is given as a premeal subcutaneous injection in patients on prandial insulin. A reduction in prandial insulin is recommended in patients with relatively good control, to avoid hypoglycemia. Weight loss of about 0.5–1.4 kg has been seen in studies.

Side-effects

- Nausea is a common side-effect, especially in the first few weeks.
- Pramlintide is contraindicated in patients with confirmed gastroparesis and hypoglycemia unawareness.

Drugs on the horizon

Sodium–glucose cotransporter 2 (SGLT2) inhibitors

- Plasma glucose is normally filtered in the renal glomeruli and then reabsorbed via sodium-dependent glucose cotransporters (SGLTs) in the proximal tubules, mostly through SGLT type 2. By inhibiting SGLT2, glucose reabsorption is decreased, glucosuria is promoted, and plasma glucose levels are decreased.
- Dapagliflozin is one such drug in this class. In clinical studies, dapagliflozin in doses of 2.5–10 mg reduced HbA1c by 0.58–0.89% when used alone, by 0.67–0.84% when used with metformin, and by 0.74–0.93% when used with insulin. In these dose ranges and combinations, hypoglycemia was reported in around 2–4% of patients.
  - ◇ In one study, the rate of hypoglycemia was 56.6% in patients on insulin plus dapagliflozin as compared to 51.8% in patients on insulin plus placebo.
- Urinary tract infections are one of the often-cited concerns for this class of drugs; the frequency has been reported to be about 5–7% in the first year, falling thereafter.

Insulin treatment

Overview

◆ Insulin is found in every vertebrate.
◆ The active part of the molecule shows few differences between species:
   ◇ Beef insulin differs from human insulin by three amino acid residues and readily induces antibody formation.
   ◇ Pork insulin, which differs by only one amino acid residue, is relatively nonimmunogenic.
   ◇ Human insulin is rarely immunogenic.
◆ The aim of insulin therapy is to mimic insulin action in patients who have a relative or absolute insulin deficiency.

Therapeutic insulin

Regular (or soluble) insulin
◆ Animal insulins are still used widely in developing countries but have been now largely replaced elsewhere by biosynthetic human insulin.
◆ Human insulin is produced by adding a DNA sequence coding for proinsulin to cultured yeast or bacterial cells. Proinsulin is subsequently enzymatically cleaved to insulin.

◆ Soluble human or animal insulins have a similar pharmacodynamic profile, entering the circulation slowly, reaching a peak 2–3 hours after injection, and predisposing to hypoglycemia due to persistent action several hours later.
   ◇ This profile differs from that of natural insulin (see Chapter 2).

Rapid-acting insulin analogs
◆ Insulin analogs have been manufactured in which the structure of the insulin molecule is modified to change its pharmacokinetics (**174**). Insulin lispro (Humalog), insulin aspart (Novorapid in the UK or Novolog in the US), and insulin glulisine (Apidra) have small modifications of their amino acid residues on the B-chain, enabling them to be absorbed and cleared more rapidly than soluble insulin.

174 Insulin analogs. Comparative structures of the available rapid-acting insulin analogs, showing the B-chain amino acid substitutions.

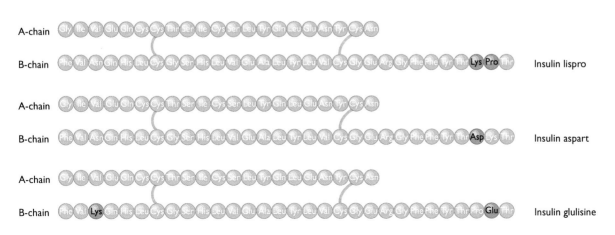

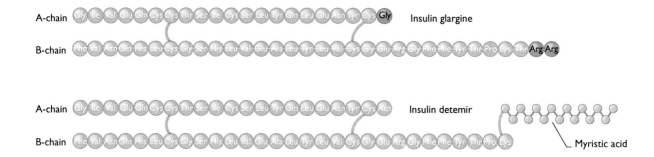

A-chain — Insulin glargine

B-chain — Arg Arg

A-chain — Insulin detemir

B-chain — Myristic acid

Insulins with prolonged action

◆ Protamine or zinc can be added to human and animal insulins to promote formation of insulin crystals, which dissolve slowly after subcutaneous injection. These insulin preparations are suspensions rather than solutions, so they are cloudy in appearance, in contrast to regular/soluble insulins and analog insulins (e.g. detemir, glargine), which are clear.

◆ NPH (neutral protamine Hagedorn) insulin, known as isophane insulin, can be premixed with soluble insulin to form stable mixtures. A range of these mixtures is available, but the combination of 30% soluble with 70% isophane is the most widely used.

◆ Zinc insulins are prepared by precipitation of insulin crystals with excess zinc, thus delaying absorption and prolonging duration of action proportional to the size of the crystals. Since an excess of zinc is present in the vial, these insulins (e.g. lente insulins including Humulin L) cannot be premixed with soluble insulin.

◆ *Insulin glargine* has its structure modified to reduce its solubility at physiological pH, thus prolonging its duration of action (**175**). It is injected as a slightly acidic (pH 4) solution and then precipitates in the tissues, which have a pH of about 7.4. The precipitates then dissolve slowly from the injection site, giving the preparation a virtually peakless action with a duration of approximately 24 hours (**176**).

175 Insulin analogs. Comparative structures of long-acting insulin analogues showing amino acid substitutions/additions. Detemir differs from human insulin in that the B30 amino acid threonine is omitted and a 14-carbon fatty acid chain – myristic acid – is attached to lysine at B29.

◆ *Insulin detemir* is another modified insulin with less peak action than the older long-acting insulins. Its prolonged action is due to hexamer stabilization, hexamer–hexamer interaction, and binding to albumin.

◆ Another very long-acting insulin – insulin degludec – is soon to be introduced. This forms soluble multihexamer assemblies after injection, resulting in an ultra-long action profile, and only needs to be injected three times a week.

◆ The longer-acting insulins that are suspensions have to be thoroughly mixed prior to subcutaneous injection to try and ensure uniform concentration in the vial. Even so, the intra-patient variability in duration and strength of action of these insulins from day to day is considerable.

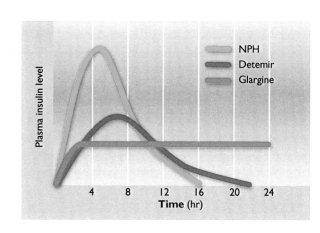

176 Insulin action profiles. Conceptual time/action profiles of the longer-acting NPH, glargine, and detemir insulins, showing duration and peaks of action.

Insulin action

	ONSET (hr)	PEAK (hr)	DURATION (hr)
Rapid- or fast-acting insulin (lispro, aspart, glulisine)	0.25–0.5	1–2	3–4
Short-acting insulin (regular)	0.5	2–3	6–8
Intermediate-acting (NPH)	1–2	4–6	8–16
Long-acting (glargine, detemir)	3–4	Generally no peak	Generally 24 hr for glargine; 9–23 hr for detemir

177 Types of insulin. These can be classed according to their pharmacodynamic characteristics: time to onset of action, time of peak action, and duration of action.

The need for injections has long been a barrier to insulin treatment in type 2 patients.

◆ In contrast, glargine and detemir have a more consistent action profile, a point commented on by many patients when they switch from one of the older insulins. Detemir, and probably glargine, is associated with less or no weight gain compared with conventional insulin treatment.

◆ These different insulins can be categorized according to the time profile of their action (**177**).
 ◇ They can also be classified according to whether they can best provide basal coverage (while the patient is in the fasting or post-absorptive state) or prandial coverage (while the patient is absorbing nutrients from meals) (see p.159).

◆ Funding agencies are concerned about the cost of insulin analogs.

Alternative insulin delivery systems
◆ There are alternative insulin delivery systems, including experimental routes:
 ◇ Inhaled insulin.
 ◇ Buccal absorbed insulin.
 ◇ Intranasal insulin.
 ◇ Implantable insulin pumps to infuse insulin intravenously or intraperitoneally.

◆ The need for injections has long been perceived as a barrier to insulin treatment in type 2 patients; it is fair to say, also, that most type 1 patients would welcome the option of insulin treatment without injections.

◆ *Inhaled insulin.* The first inhaled insulin (Exubera, Pfizer), an inhalation powder of human insulin of rDNA origin, was approved for use in 2006 but withdrawn in 2008 due to lack of commercial success.
 ◇ The time/action profile showed a similar onset to that of the subcutaneously injected rapid-acting analogs, but with a duration of action more like that of regular insulin (**178**).
 ◇ The reproducibility of action was similar to those of subcutaneous insulin injections.

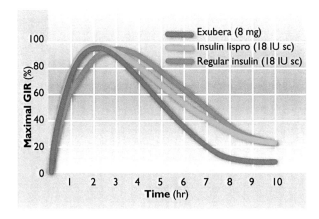

178 Inhaled insulin. Time/action profile of inhaled insulin (Exubera) compared with regular insulin and insulin lispro given subcutaneously.

Insulin treatment

- Exubera was well accepted in clinical trials of both type 1 and type 2 diabetes, achieving equivalent glycemic control when substituted for premeal subcutaneous insulin or oral agents.
  - ◇ Most trial participants expressed a preference for remaining on inhaled insulin rather than reverting to their previous regimens. However, trial participants were often patients who specifically disliked injections, so their preference was perhaps predictable.
  - ◇ When this insulin became available for everyday prescription there was a very limited 'take up', leading the manufacturer to withdraw it on commercial grounds.
  - ◇ Hypoglycemia has been the most frequent adverse event, similar in frequency to that of subcutaneous insulin. Other forms of inhaled insulin are in development.
- Safety is a vital concern. Specific concerns with inhaled insulin understandably relate to respiratory symptoms and pulmonary function.
  - ◇ Dry mouth, mild cough, and mild to moderate dyspnea all occurred more frequently than with comparator treatment in the clinical trials, but very few patients discontinued treatment because of these symptoms.
  - ◇ FEV_1 (forced expiratory volume in 1 second) decreases by a mean of 1–1.5% in the first few weeks of treatment, but thereafter stabilizes; it is recommended that all patients should have assessment of pulmonary function (spirometry) before starting inhaled insulin.
  - ◇ The treatment is not recommended for smokers, until they have quit for at least 6 months, or for patients with asthma or chronic obstructive pulmonary disease.
- Another potential concern is whether prolonged, repeated exposure of the bronchi and smaller airways to insulin would promote the formation of granulomatous or mitotic disease.
  - ◇ It has been reported that a small number of subjects who received Exubera in the initial clinical trials have subsequently been diagnosed with lung cancer. The numbers do not reach statistical significance when compared with control subjects in the same trials, but this will, no doubt, increase fears about the long-term safety of inhaled insulin.

- *Insulin spray.* An insulin spray (Oral-Lyn, Generex) which delivers human insulin for absorption through the buccal mucous membrane, but not the lungs, has been approved for commercial marketing and prescription since 2005 in various countries (but not Europe or North America).
  - ◇ The peak insulin concentration occurs about 25 minutes after administration, with onset of action occurring a little later and peaking at about 45 minutes. There have been no post-marketing reports of this buccal insulin's long-term use.
- The intranasal route and the implantable pumps for intraperitoneal/intravenous insulin delivery are still under investigation.

Indications for insulin treatment

- In classical childhood- or adolescent-onset type 1 diabetes the need for insulin treatment is clear and unequivocal.
- When autoimmune diabetes develops later in life the extent of insulin deficiency is initially less severe. Patients are commonly misdiagnosed as having type 2 diabetes, but many, though by no means all, progress to insulin treatment.
- In type 2 diabetes there are no absolutes. There is no *a priori* reason not to use insulin as an initial therapy in type 2 diabetes, but few physicians recommend that. Insulin treatment is generally recommended when the other alternatives have failed to achieve adequate glycemic control.
  - ◇ Many type 2 patients will at some stage benefit from insulin treatment as a part of their routine treatment.
  - ◇ We have traditionally been too slow in confronting the need for insulin in our patients, due to a combination of patient anxiety about insulin treatment and clinical inertia.

Many type 2 patients will benefit from insulin therapy as a part of their routine treatment.

- Other situations where insulin is accepted as 'the treatment of choice' for the type 2 diabetic, or hyperglycemic, patient include:
  - ◇ Pregnancy, when diet therapy alone is not sufficient (though there is a growing literature indicating that some oral agents may be quite safe and effective).
  - ◇ Intercurrent illness, especially infections.
  - ◇ Myocardial infarction.
  - ◇ Surgical (and, with qualification, medical) intensive-care patients.
  - ◇ Hyperosmolar nonketotic coma (HONK).
- Decisions to be made about insulin treatment include:
  - ◇ Type of insulin.
  - ◇ Timing of injections.
  - ◇ Dose of insulin.
  - ◇ Education regarding adjustment of insulin dose.
  - ◇ Need for assistance.
  - ◇ Blood glucose monitoring.
  - ◇ Education regarding hypoglycemia.
  - ◇ Need to carry glucose.
  - ◇ Additional cost of insulin analogs.

Insulin regimen: type 1 diabetes

- To establish an insulin regimen, a typical day can be considered to comprise periods of basal insulin production – essentially the fasting and postabsorptive states – interspersed with bursts of prandial and postprandial insulin production.
- In healthy individuals, with normal glucose tolerance and taking three meals a day, basal insulin accounts for about 50% of the total. This will naturally be modified by physical activity and normal diurnal fluctuations in counter-regulatory hormone production. Mealtime or prandial insulin makes up the other 50% of insulin secretion. Secretion of insulin in response to meals is rapid, with a relatively narrow peak, and results in absorption of glucose in tissues, with excess glucose being stored as glycogen in the liver and muscle or converted to lipid.
- While it makes sense to mimic this pattern, there is no rule when it comes to the best regimen, which should be tailored to suit individual needs (**179**).

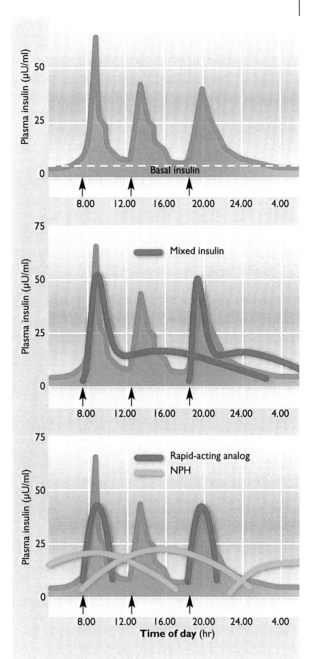

179 **Insulin regimens.** The pattern of physiological basal–bolus insulin secretion (top), with peak action at mealtimes (arrows), can be mimicked by therapy schedules. These can use both rapid-acting and longer-acting (NPH) insulin or mixed (rapid/longer-acting) insulin or a single injection of long-acting insulin with rapid-acting insulin at mealtimes.

Insulin treatment

- Regimens with multiple injections (**180**) are more flexible, and the risk of hypoglycemia can be reduced by using long-acting insulin with minimal peak action for basal needs and rapid-acting insulin analogs for mealtime coverage.
- The closest we can get to mimicking physiological insulin production (apart from pancreas or islet cell transplantation) is with continuous subcutaneous insulin infusion (CSII) pumps (**181**). CSII could be suggested for most patients with type 1 diabetes, but specific reasons include:
  - ◇ Poor metabolic control with hyperglycemia.
  - ◇ Poor metabolic control with hypoglycemia.
  - ◇ Instability of metabolic control with swings from high to low glucose.
  - ◇ Patients who have a significant dawn phenomenon (a rise in blood glucose in the early hours) – since a pump can deliver insulin at different rates or doses at different times of the day.
- For a period (weeks to months) after type 1 diabetes has been diagnosed, there will usually be some residual endogenous insulin secretion and less intensive insulin regimens may achieve excellent glycemic control at that time.
  - ◇ Occasionally, insulin treatment can be temporarily withdrawn and blood glucose levels will remain normal. This 'remission' of diabetes is popularly referred to as the 'honeymoon period' and it is important to emphasize to patients that it is, regrettably, a temporary phenomenon.

Common insulin regimens

A single daily subcutaneous injection of long-acting insulin (in patients with type 2 diabetes)

Two daily injections of premixed fast-acting and intermediate-duration insulins

Four daily injections: three of fast-acting insulin given with each meal and one intermediate or long-acting insulin at bedtime

A subcutaneous infusion of fast-acting insulin given via a pump throughout the day

180 Insulin regimens. It is important to match the choice of regimen to the clinical and lifesetyle needs of the patient.

- Once the honeymoon period is over, patients with type 1 diabetes who have a relatively normal body weight will typically require a daily insulin dose of between 0.5 and 1.0 IU/kg.
- The precise distribution of the insulin dosages will depend on a number of factors.
- If the basal coverage is supplied by an insulin like glargine or detemir that effectively has no peak, then it is reasonable to apportion approximately 50% of the total daily dose to that.
  - ◇ For glargine, this can usually be given as a single injection at approximately the same time each day, usually at bedtime, but chosen to fit in with the individual's lifestyle.
  - ◇ In some people – particularly adolescents and young adults – with irregular work and leisure schedules, it may make more sense to split the glargine insulin dose in two to ensure 'round the clock' coverage.
  - ◇ In a small percentage of patients, insulin glargine may not last the full 24 hours, making a split-dose regimen more effective.
- If the basal component is supplied by a long-acting insulin that does have a significant peak – such as isophane/NPH – then that insulin will make a significant contribution to mealtime coverage as well as basal requirements, so that proportionately more basal and less prandial insulin will comprise the total dose.
  - ◇ Insulin detemir probably lies somewhere between glargine and isophane/NPH in this respect, and both detemir and isophane/NPH (plus in selected cases glargine) can be given twice a day when used as basal insulin in type 1 diabetes.

Continuous subcutaneous insulin infusion: insulin pump treatment

- CSII at low levels in the fasting and postabsorptive states, coupled with mealtime increases, represents an attempt to mimic normal pancreatic β-cell function that can realistically be offered to many, if not most, people with type 1 diabetes.
- Since the pioneering days in the 1970s of bulky, makeshift pumps, advances in microchip technology have led to the development and availability of quite sophisticated devices that are small enough to be concealed in clothing or 'worn' like a pager or mobile phone (**182**).

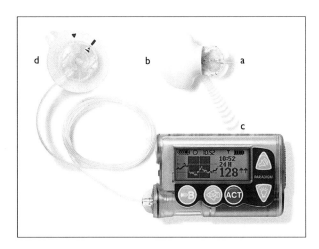

181 CSII. In this sensor-augmented system, a sensor (a) attached to a transmitter (b) communicates with the pump (c), which delivers insulin via a cannula to the infusion set (d).

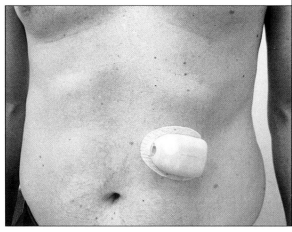

182 CSII. A tubeless, waterproof insulin pump in a patient with type 1 diabetes. This device ataches directly to the skin via a cannula and is managed by a wireless pocket computer.

◆ Insulin is fed to the subcutaneous tissue from a reservoir via a fine flexible catheter that is easily inserted by the patient; this catheter is changed every 2 or 3 days.
  ◇ With careful attention to simple hygiene, and relocation of the infusion site each time, there are very few problems with infection or other local adverse effects, such as fibrosis or lipo-hypertrophy.
◆ There is general consensus that a rapid-acting insulin analog rather than soluble human insulin works best in the pump.
◆ Pumps can be programmed to alter the basal rate of infusion many times during a 24-hour period:
  ◇ Some patients find that a single basal rate over 24 hours works well.
  ◇ Many patients do better with basal rates that take account of such things as diurnal changes in counter-regulatory hormones, work patterns, and regular exercise.
  ◇ The most sophisticated pumps offer the ability to set alternative basal regimens on specific days to accommodate, for example, the demands of shift work or change of activity at weekends compared to weekdays.
◆ It is rare that basal rates greater than 1 IU/h are required, and many patients require considerably less; this has to be worked out on an individual basis. Advice from an experienced diabetes educator and 'pump trainer' can be invaluable.

◆ Although patients can effectively 'forget about the pump' so far as basal insulin delivery is concerned once the settings are in place, the same is not true of mealtime insulin boluses. Pumps do not yet have sufficient technological sophistication to anticipate and respond to the increased insulin needs that accompany eating, so the success or failure of pump therapy can rest on the individual's preparedness to manage mealtime insulin.
  ◇ Modern pumps do offer programs that help calculate the appropriate dose in relation to the composition of the meal, and the choice of delivering the mealtime insulin as a single bolus or a 'square wave' delivery over a defined period, or a combination of the two.
  ◇ This aspect of insulin pump therapy still requires as much active input from the patient as any insulin injection regimen, and for this reason it should not be assumed that pump treatment will necessarily lead to better glucose control.
  ◇ Several studies confirm that forgetting, or neglecting, to deliver a mealtime bolus is one of the commonest problems among (particularly younger) pump-treated patients.

Insulin treatment

183 Advantages of CSII. As well as delivering insulin in a more physiologically precise manner than injections, pump therapy also offers greater flexibility.

◆ It is very important to educate patients that, because this type of insulin delivery does not involve the build-up of a subcutaneous depot of insulin, development of ketoacidosis will occur rapidly in the event of system malfunction, such as blockage of the catheter.

◇ Patients can swing from a state of normo-glycemia to severe, and life-threatening, ketoacidosis in as little as 4–6 hours.

◇ This has been seen occasionally when a patient disconnects the pump to have a shower or a short swim, forgetting to reconnect it afterwards; waterproof pumps are now available (see **182**).

◆ So far there have been relatively few randomized studies comparing pumps with intensive injection therapy, and most of those predated the availabilty of long-acting 'basal' insulin analogs (glargine and detemir).

◇ 'Before and after' studies generally show that HbA1c can be expected to improve when a patient with inadequate control switches from intensive treatment with injections to CSII, and several such reports emphasize that, particularly for patients who remain on pump therapy for more than 1 year, the improvement in HbA1c can be substantial.

◇ In the absence of well-designed randomized trials using short- and long-acting analog insulin as comparator, it is difficult to attribute such improvements solely to the pump technology – enthusiasm of both patients and providers (particularly in the US) for the technology, plus education, obviously plays an important role.

Ketoacidosis will occur rapidly if the pump malfunctions or a catheter is blocked.

Potential advantages of CSII

Decreased variability of insulin absorption

Greater ability to cover snacks as well as main meals

Greater flexibility with meals and snacks

Decreased risk of nocturnal hypoglycemia

Greater ability to counteract 'dawn' phenomenon

Ability to adjust for exercise

Lack of subcutaneous depot of insulin decreases risk of exercise-induced hypoglycemia

◆ There are several reasons for thinking that CSII should provide better glycemic control than intensive injection therapy (**183**).

◆ Many nonrandomized studies suggest that even if pump therapy does not inevitably lead to a lower HbA1c it will enable a near-normal HbA1c to be achieved with less risk of hypoglycemia than will intensive-injection regimens, though the use of insulin analogs, especially for basal coverage, has reduced the risk of severe hypoglycemia.

◆ Theoretically, there is no reason why every type 1 diabetic patient should not be offered the option of pump treatment. However, the costs (pump plus catheter supplies) are greater than those of injection treatment, and this is a limiting factor.

◇ If, in the future, it becomes clear that improved pump technology leads almost invariably to better glycemic control and a reduced risk of diabetic complications, then the long-term cost-effectiveness may lead to a great increase in its use.

◆ At present, it is difficult to say that there is any specific situation that warrants pump treatment over injections.

◇ Patient choice, within the cost constraints of the prevailing healthcare system, is probably still the most common deciding factor.

◇ Pregnancy is one situation where many centers will offer pump treatment.

◇ Arguments that pumps may not be suitable for children may apply only to the very young, bearing in mind the ease with which children and adolescents readily master all sorts of microchip devices.

Implantable glucose monitors

◆ Frequent and consistent self-monitoring of blood glucose is essential to the success of pump therapy.

◆ Concurrent with advances in pump technology there has been development of accurate and reliable 'real-time' sensor devices for glucose levels in interstitial fluid obtained either subcutaneously or percutaneously.

◆ Such devices give results that correlate well with laboratory-measured plasma glucose, but they are expensive and the sensors have to be replaced frequently. However, further refinement, coupled with the increasing sophistication of wireless communication between devices, could eventually 'close the loop' between prevailing blood glucose and insulin delivery.

◆ Implantable monitors may be used with insulin injections and can be especially helpful in identifying unrecognized hypoglycemia.

Insulin regimen: type 2 diabetes

General considerations

◆ Insulin treatment in type 2 diabetes is most often prescribed when treatment with oral agents has been insufficient, though there is no reason why insulin could not be considered from the time of diagnosis.

◆ Starting patients with type 2 diabetes on insulin has long been hedged around with fears, anxieties, and misunderstanding on the part of patients and physicians. Numerous reasons have been put forward for failure to get patients on to insulin when glycemic control is clearly inadequate despite maximal doses of oral agents.

◇ It is understandable that most patients will prefer not to take injections if other satisfactory alternatives are available; the idea that insulin treatment represents any failure on the patient's part should be avoided.

◇ Too often the 'threat' of insulin treatment is brandished as a means of achieving better compliance with diet, exercise, and oral agents; this is not just bad psychology – it fails to appreciate that many patients, simply through the nature of the condition, will remain hyperglycemic despite reasonable adherence to prescribed regimens.

◆ A more appropriate approach is to emphasize at the outset that insulin deficiency is an integral part of type 2 diabetes and that, therefore, many patients will require and benefit from insulin treatment at some time.

◆ Because type 2 diabetes so often affects several family members and generations, many patients recount hearing of some relative who seemed to be fine until he or she received insulin late in the stage of the disease, after which there was steady deterioration.

◆ Physicians and other health carers may also still entertain notions that insulin treatment, by leading to hyperinsulinism, increases the risk of atherosclerosis. Both UKPDS and the DIGAMI Study have effectively dispelled this myth:

◇ In the UKPDS, insulin treatment was no more likely than diet or sulfonylurea therapy to be associated with cardiovascular events in a diabetic population that was essentially free of clinical cardiovascular disease at study entry.

◇ In the DIGAMI Study, diabetic patients had a better outcome following acute myocardial infarction if insulin was substituted for oral agents during hospitalization (and beyond in many cases).

◆ Modern disposable syringes and pen devices with ultra-fine needles now make injection virtually atraumatic (**184**).

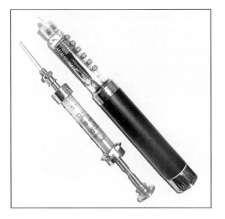

184 Insulin pen compared with traditional syringe.
Insulin pens can be either disposable (prefilled) or durable (with replaceable cartridges).

Insulin treatment

◆ Positive expectations of benefit can outweigh reservations about insulin self-injection (extending to needle phobia, hypoglycemia, and weight gain). This was amply demonstrated by the relative welcome that many patients gave when offered a trial of the noninsulin injectable exenatide because of expectations that it would promote weight loss.

◆ Any insulin treatment brings with it a risk of hypoglycemia, but risk of severe hypoglycemia is considerably less in patients with type 2 diabetes than in those with type 1 diabetes.

   ◇ This may be due partly to increased insulin resistance, and regimens that employ supplementation of basal insulin in the absence of mealtime dosing are also less likely to cause severe hypoglycemia.

◆ Given that hypoglycemia is an unpleasant and potentially serious adverse effect of insulin, it makes sense to start with low doses that will be unlikely to cause hypoglycemia, and gradually increase the dose thereafter; this is true whatever insulin regimen is selected in type 2 diabetes.

◆ There are two components to the insulin-secretory defect in type 2 diabetes: fasting insulin and first-phase insulin response.

   ◇ Loss of first-phase insulin response to ingested food is, perhaps, the earliest abnormality, and this defect is apparent in subjects with fasting glucose levels higher than normal but not yet at the level of 7 mmol/l (126 mg/dl) which defines diabetes.

   ◇ In these individuals, and also those with recently diagnosed type 2 diabetes, the fasting serum insulin level often appears similar to, or even higher than, fasting insulin levels in normal subjects, as insulin deficiency is relative to the higher glucose level and, in effect, at an early stage there is a defect in both mealtime as well as basal insulin secretion.

◆ The choice of insulin treatment could, therefore, lie between augmenting basal and mealtime insulin levels, or a combination of the two. Consideration of the typical 24-hour glucose profile in type 2 diabetes is useful in this respect (**185**).

   ◇ The *major* abnormality is that the elevated fasting glucose results in the entire glucose profile shifting upwards; the postprandial glucose excursions are greater in diabetes, and increase as the fasting glucose increases.

   ◇ The entire area under the profile represents the integrated glucose, corresponding to HbA1c level; augmenting basal insulin and reducing the fasting glucose towards normal – effectively shifting the whole line downwards – should lead to a greater overall reduction in glycemia and HbA1c than targeting only the postprandial glucose peaks by giving mealtime insulin.

   ◇ Fasting and postprandial glucose are not independent variables, however, and action taken to specifically change the one will have a 'knock-on' effect on the other, so either strategy can be expected to have success, and an ideal strategy would be to target both.

   ◇ At this stage, patient choice, convenience, and economics come into play.

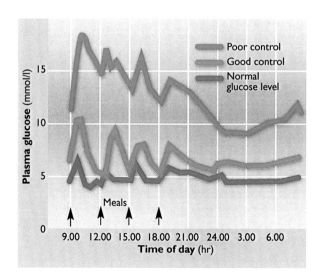

185 24-hour glucose profile. As plasma glucose falls from high towards normal levels, so the basal glucose falls and is an indicator of glucose control. *Adapted from Holman RR and Turner RC, 1981.*

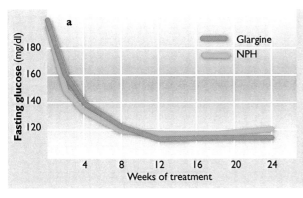

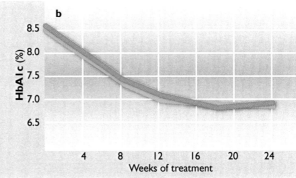

Basal insulin

◆ Isophane or NPH insulin at bedtime has been shown to be an effective means of reducing fasting glucose and HbA1c in patients treated with metformin or sulfonylurea as oral mono-therapy, or metformin and sulfonylurea as dual oral therapy.

◇ The insulin action overnight has the effect of limiting hepatic glucose output, leading to improved fasting glucose.

◇ Isophane/NPH insulin has a significant peak of action some 4–6 hours after subcutaneous injection, so there is a significant risk of nocturnal hypoglycemia, which, however, is usually mild.

◆ A truly basal insulin is one which would have little or no peak action; insulin glargine and detemir are the only currently available preparations that meet this requirement.

◇ A comparison between isophane/NPH and glargine as basal insulin treatment in type 2 diabetes found them to be equally effective in reducing fasting glucose and HbA1c (**186**); nocturnal hypoglycemia occurred approximately twice as frequently with isophane/NPH as with glargine, though there was a small increase in daytime hypoglycemia with glargine (**187**).

◇ In one study of patients treated with either metformin or sulfonylurea or both, glargine was also given: at the end of the study the mean HbA1c was just under 7% (53 mmol/mol), from a starting HbA1c of 8.7% (72 mmol/mol).

A truly basal insulin has little or no peak action.

---

186 Basal insulin treatment. Insulin glargine had similar effects on fasting glucose (a) and HbA1c (b) in the Treat-to-Target trial. Insulin dosages were titrated upwards on a weekly basis, depending on the fasting glucose level. *Adapted from Riddle MC, Rosenstock J, et al.*

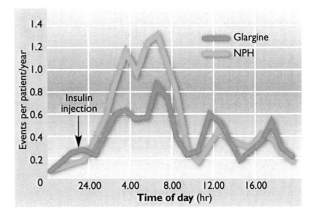

187 Hypoglycemic events. Although both glargine and NPH achieved similar fasting glucose and HbA1c levels in the Treat-to-Target trial, glargine did so with markedly less nocturnal hypoglycemia. *Adapted from Riddle MC, Rosenstock J, et al.*

◆ Detemir, which has significantly less peak action than NPH but not as 'flat' a profile as glargine or as long a half-life, is another alternative.

◆ Basal insulin supplementation of existing oral regimens that have failed to achieve a satisfactory HbA1c is now the most common pathway for the introduction of insulin treatment in type 2 diabetes. This typically occurs after the patient has been on a combination of two or three oral agents, but it can be applied also when oral monotherapy does not result in a satisfactory HbA1c.

Insulin treatment

- The ADA/EASD consensus treatment guidelines make the point that insulin is potentially the most effective 'next step' after monotherapy fails to achieve the goal.
- A single injection each day is easily accepted by most patients when the potential benefits are explained to them. Administering the first injection during the course of a routine clinic visit often convinces even reluctant patients of the ease of the treatment.
  - ◇ With insulin glargine the timing of subsequent injections can be selected by the patient to fit in best with their daily routine and preferences. Many choose to give the injection first thing in the morning, while others prefer dinner time or bedtime; the important thing is consistency from day to day.
  - ◇ With isophane/NPH and insulin detemir bedtime injection is preferable.
- Regardless of which particular insulin is selected, it makes sense to start with a relatively low dose that would not be expected to cause hypoglycemia, and then to titrate the dose gradually but steadily, aiming ideally for fasting glucose levels persistently in the range of 4–7 mmol/l (about 70–130 mg/dl).
  - ◇ This needs to be explained and frequently reinforced to patients, who will often become concerned that the strategy may not be working if, after a few weeks of steadily increasing insulin dosage, the fasting glucose is still not at goal.
- Because of the insulin resistance in type 2 diabetes the effective dose of basal insulin can seem alarmingly high to patients; experience suggests that patients start to get concerned when the dose exceeds 30–40 IU.
  - ◇ It is therefore imperative that patients learn that there is no predetermined 'maximum dose' of insulin, and that some patients require much higher doses, sometimes well over 100 IU per day as a single injection, for this regimen to be successful.

- There is no single 'dosage algorithm' that is necessarily better than another. Some studies have used 10 IU, or 0.5 IU/kg, or 0.1 IU/kg (young children) as a starting dose, with increases made weekly on the basis of the mean fasting glucose, while others recommend more frequent dose increases, such as an additional single unit every day until the 'target' fasting glucose is being achieved fairly consistently. The important thing is for the patient to recognize the need for insulin adjustment and to participate in the process.
- This strategy enables many patients to achieve HbA1c levels of <7% (IFCC 53 mmol/mol), but inevitably some patients will start experiencing hypoglycemia, either nocturnal or daytime, before the target fasting glucose has been achieved.
  - ◇ In that case the dose of the basal insulin should be reduced to eliminate the hypoglycemia, and additional treatment – mealtime insulin, exenatide or perhaps a gliptin – will be required.
  - ◇ It should be noted that addition of a gliptin in a patient on basal insulin treatment is not (yet) approved by the regulatory authorities, but it is quite commonly done in the UK and US and can be effective.

Mealtime insulin
- Targeting the postprandial rise in glucose is another potential means of improving all-round glycemia.
- Epidemiological studies suggest that postprandial glucose is a greater determinant of cardiovascular risk than fasting glucose, so there is a school of thought that it makes more sense to train our guns primarily on postprandial hyperglycemia.
- The need for several injections per day makes this option less attractive as an initial insulin treatment for most type 2 patients, though it can be successful in those who try it.

It is important for the patient to recognize the need for insulin and participate actively in the process.

188 Premixed biphasic insulin. In patients with type 2 diabetes poorly controlled on oral antidiabetic drugs, initiating insulin therapy with twice-daily 70% NPH/30% aspart (BIAsp 70/30) was more effective in achieving HbA1c targets than once-daily glargine. *Adapted from Raskin P, Allen E, et al.*

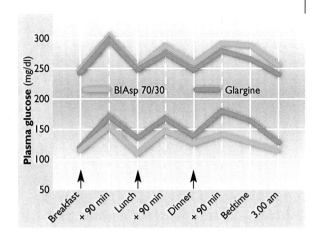

Premixed insulin

◆ Premixed 'fixed ratio' insulin, consisting of rapid-acting or soluble insulin plus isophane/NPH, is a convenient way of trying to provide both basal and mealtime insulin supplementation.
 ◇ The most commonly used fixed ratios are 30/70% soluble and isophane/NPH or 25/75% rapid-acting/NPH.
◆ The obvious attraction is the convenience of having both components in one premixed syringe or pen device, and injections are typically given before breakfast and before the evening meal.
◆ A randomized study comparing this approach (using an aspart and isophane/NPH mixture) with once-daily insulin glargine showed this to be successful in terms of reducing HbA1c, and there is a particular benefit in lowering the postprandial glucose after the evening meal (**188**).
 ◇ A potential drawback is that this type of regimen tends to sometimes give more insulin than needed, with the pre-evening meal injection heightening the risk of nocturnal hypoglycemia even in comparison to bedtime isophane/NPH (see **179**).
 ◇ A defect of the study was that on adding insulin treatment all patients discontinued sulfonylurea, while continuing whatever metformin and/or TZD treatment they were taking. It is arguable that patients randomized to glargine, without the possible 'mealtime boost' of sulfonylurea, were thus disadvantaged. Not surprisingly, there was more hypoglycemia in patients treated with premixed insulin than with glargine.
◆ As with the single injection of basal insulin, it makes sense to start with relatively low doses of fixed-ratio insulin, and gradually and steadily increase the doses until the required level of control is achieved or hypoglycemia occurs.

Metabolic instability on insulin

◆ There are several factors surrounding insulin use that might affect glucose control.
◆ Errors in insulin injection technique:
 ◇ The wrong dose or timing.
 ◇ Air in the syringe.
 ◇ Poor injection technique.
◆ Alterations in insulin pharmacokinetics:
 ◇ Injection into the wrong place (e.g. into area of lipohypertrophy or intradermal or intramuscular injection) (common) (**189**).

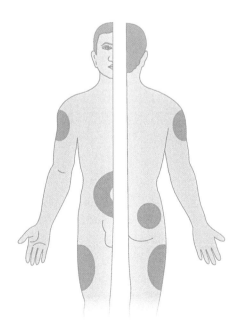

189 Insulin injection sites. Injections should usually be made into the subcutaneous tissue. The abdomen has the fastest rate of absorption, followed by the arms, thighs, and buttocks.

◇ Anti-insulin antibodies bind insulin (rare) (**190**).

◇ Insulin clearance is rapid (rare).

◆ Alterations in insulin action:

◇ Insulin receptor defects.

◇ Insulin postreceptor defects (e.g. obesity, type 2 diabetes).

◇ Drugs.

◇ Counter-regulatory hormone disturbances.

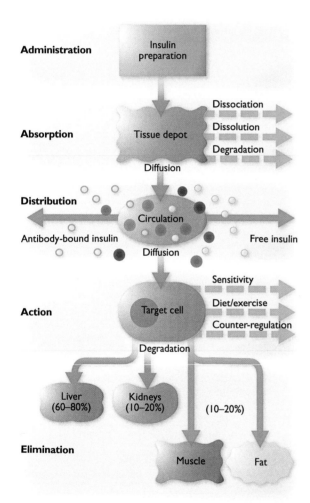

Administration — Insulin preparation

Absorption — Tissue depot — Dissociation / Dissolution / Degradation

Diffusion

Distribution — Circulation — Antibody-bound insulin — Free insulin

Diffusion

Action — Target cell — Sensitivity / Diet/exercise / Counter-regulation

Degradation

Elimination — Liver (60–80%) — Kidneys (10–20%) — (10–20%) — Muscle — Fat

190 Insulin pharmacokinetics. The main steps comprise absorption, distribution – including binding to circulating insulin antibodies, if present, or to insulin receptors – and, ultimately, degradation and excretion through a variety of processes. Insulin action is determined by the sensitivity of the patient to insulin, amount of exercise, diet, and the various counter-regulatory mechanisms that prevail.

Complications: hypoglycemia

◆ Hypoglycemia is a common problem in patients on insulin treatment, and to a lesser extent in patients treated with insulin secretagogues.

◇ In the DCCT there was an inverse relationship between HbA1c level and severe hypoglycemia. Diabetes control is thus a compromise between risk of hypoglycemia and risk of diabetes complications (**191**).

◆ Hypoglycemia is potentially the greatest barrier to achieving normoglycemia.

◆ Virtually all insulin-treated patients experience intermittent symptoms of hypoglycemia, and approximately 10% will have a severe episode requiring assistance each year. A small minority suffer attacks that are so frequent and severe as to be virtually disabling.

◆ Hypoglycemia results from an imbalance between injected insulin or oral hypoglycemic therapy and a patient's normal diet, activity, and metabolic requirements.

◇ For patients on insulin, the times of greatest risk are before meals and during the night.

◇ Patients on secretagogues are at greatest risk during the late afternoon.

◇ Irregular eating habits, unusual exertion, and alcohol excess may precipitate episodes.

◇ Some cases in those on insulin therapy appear to be due simply to variation in insulin absorption.

◆ Symptoms of hypoglycemia develop when the blood glucose level falls towards 3.5 mmol/l (60–70 mg/dl) and typically develop over a few minutes (**192**).

◆ Common symptoms include altered mental alertness, hunger, feeling shaky, and distortion of vision, while physical signs include 'adrenergic' features of pallor, sweating, tremor, and a pounding heart beat (**193**).

◇ Patients progressing to more severe hypoglycemia appear pale, drowsy or detached – signs that their relatives quickly learn to recognize.

Hypoglycemia is potentially the greatest barrier to achieving normoglycemia.

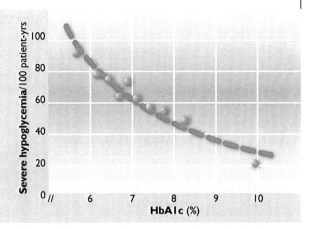

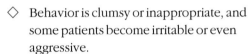

191 Hypoglycemia and low HbA1c. Rates of retinopathy (a) and severe hypoglycemia (b) relative to HbA1c level. The risk of hypoglycemia needs to be balanced against that of other complications. *Adapted from DCCT Research Group data.*

◇ Behavior is clumsy or inappropriate, and some patients become irritable or even aggressive.
◇ Some such patients slip rapidly into hypoglycemic coma.
◇ Occasionally, patients develop convulsions during hypoglycemic coma, especially at night. It is important not to confuse this with idiopathic epilepsy, especially since patients with frequent hypoglycemia often show EEG abnormalities.
◇ Another presentation is with a hemiparesis that resolves within a few minutes when glucose is administered.

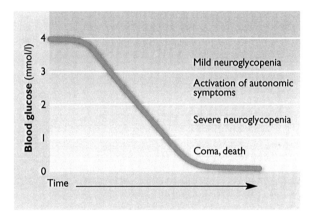

192 Development of hypoglycemia. Glycemic thresholds for release of epinephrine and subsequent activation of autonomic and neuroglycopenic symptoms.

193 Hypoglycemia symptoms. Awareness of symptoms and timely intervention can avoid a hypoglycemic event.

Common signs and symptoms of hypoglycemia and actions to be taken by the patient

SYMPTOMS	PHYSIOLOGICAL MECHANISM	BLOOD GLUCOSE AT ONSET (mmol/l[mg/dl])	INTERVENTION REQUIRED
Hunger, sweating, tremor, palpitations	Autonomic response to subnormal glycemia	Below ≈3.5 [63]	Take glucose-rich sweets, drink or food
Cognitive dysfunction, atypical behavior, speech difficulty, uncoordination, dizziness, drowsiness	Neuroglycopenia (brain deprived of glucose)	Below ≈2.8 [50]	Take glucose-rich sweets, drink or food; seek assistance
Malaise, headache, nausea, reduced consciousness	Severe neuroglycopenia	Below ≈2.0 [36]	Third-party intervention required
Convulsions, coma	Severe neuroglycopenia	Below ≈1.5 [27]	Medical intervention essential

Insulin treatment

Hypoglycemic unawareness

◆ Many patients with long-standing insulin-treated diabetes report loss of these warning symptoms and are at a greater risk of progressing to more severe hypoglycemia.

◆ This is rarely a problem until diabetes has been present for a number of years. People with diabetes have an impaired ability to counter-regulate glucose levels after hypoglycemia.

◇ The glucagon response is invariably deficient, even though the α cells are preserved and respond normally to other stimuli.

◇ The epinephrine response may also fail in patients with a long duration of diabetes, and this is associated with loss of warning symptoms.

◇ Recurrent hypoglycemia may itself induce a state of hypoglycemia unawareness (**194**). The ability to recognize the condition may sometimes be restored by relaxing control for a few weeks.

Nocturnal hypoglycemia

◆ This is a major cause of anxiety for patients and relatives – particularly parents of children and adolescents with type 1 diabetes. Common experience suggests that nocturnal hypoglycemia, and the thought of falling asleep never to reawaken, hold particular terror for some patients and for many parents.

◆ Basal insulin requirements fall during the night but increase again from about 4 am onwards, at a time when levels of injected insulin are falling. As a result many patients awake with high blood glucose levels, but find that injecting more insulin at night increases the risk of hypoglycemia in the early hours of the morning.

◆ Use of newer insulin analogs like insulin glargine, which effectively is without a 'peak' effect, and detemir, which has a considerably smaller peak than, for example isophane/NPH, has been shown to reduce the likelihood of nocturnal hypoglycemia by about 50% compared with other intermediate- or long-acting insulins.

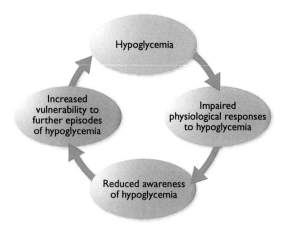

194 Hypoglycemic unawareness. Lack of warning symptoms, or a failure to recognize them, can lead to a vicious circle of repeated hypoglycemia.

◆ Other strategies that will help to minimize the likelihood of nocturnal hypoglycemia include:

◇ Checking that a bedtime snack is taken regularly.

◇ For patients taking twice-daily mixed insulin to separate their evening dose and take the intermediate insulin at bedtime rather than before supper.

◇ Reducing the dose of soluble insulin before supper, since the effects of this persist well into the night.

◇ Changing patients on a multiple injection regimen with soluble insulin to a rapid-acting insulin analog.

Recurrent severe hypoglycemia

◆ Each year about 10% of patients on insulin will have an episode of severe hypoglycemia requiring intervention by someone else.

◇ About 1–3% of patients with type 1 diabetes have recurrent severe hypoglycemia.

◇ Most patients with recurrent persistent problems are adults who have had diabetes for more than 10 years with low production of endogenous insulin as estimated by C-peptide.

◆ Pancreatic α cells are still present in undiminished numbers, but their glucagon response to hypoglycemia is virtually absent and the catecholamine response may be impaired. These patients therefore lack a major component of the hormonal defense against hypoglycemia.

- The following factors predispose to recurrent hypoglycemia:
  - ◇ Overtreatment with insulin. Frequent hypoglycemia impairs the response to further hypoglycemia within 2 weeks and lowers the blood glucose level at which symptoms develop.
  - ◇ Endocrine causes, including pituitary insufficiency, adrenal insufficiency, hypothyroidism, and premenstrual insulin sensitivity.
  - ◇ Gastrointestinal causes, including exocrine pancreatic failure, celiac disease, and diabetic gastroparesis.
  - ◇ Renal failure. The kidneys are important for the clearance of insulin and oral hypoglycemics, such as sulfonylureas, and also contribute to gluconeogenesis, which diminishes with declining renal function.
  - ◇ Patients may manipulate their therapy or misunderstand it.
  - ◇ Alcohol use has been implicated in up to 19% of severe hypoglycemic episodes. Alcohol in excess will suppress hepatic gluconeogenesis and, particularly if taken late in the evening, the effect may coincide with the nocturnal decline in cortisol, predisposing the patient to severe nocturnal hypoglycemia.
  - ◇ Other 'recreational' drug use. In a recent report, 10% of diabetic patients under the age of 50 tested positive for illicit drugs at the time of a severe hypoglycemic episode.

Treating hypoglycemia

- Treatment depends on the severity of the hypoglycemia.
- If it is practical to do so, it is useful to confirm the diagnosis with a blood or plasma glucose estimation by finger-stick. However, if hypoglycemia may reasonably be assumed, it is important not to delay treatment simply because of lack of absolute certainty about the diagnosis.
  - ◇ Administering treatment for hypoglycemia when in fact hypoglycemia is not present is potentially less harmful than delaying treatment to someone who is truly hypoglycemic, as long as there is adequate assessment and follow-up over several hours.

- All patients and their close relatives and friends should learn about the risks of hypoglycemia and to recognize and treat the symptoms.
- Patients should be warned that taking excessive carbohydrate could be counterproductive, since this may cause rebound hyperglycemia; however, in practice it is notoriously difficult to avoid some degree of overcorrection.
- The dangers of alcohol excess and of hypoglycemia while driving need to be emphasized.

Mild hypoglycemia

- Any form of rapidly absorbed carbohydrate will relieve the early symptoms, and sufferers should always carry glucose or sweets.
  - ◇ Drowsy individuals will be able to take carbohydrate (15 g) in liquid form (e.g. Lucozade).
  - ◇ It is also sensible to recommend a small amount of less readily absorbed carbohydrate (30 g), particularly when an oral hypoglycemic drug or longer-acting insulin is implicated as a cause of the hypoglycemia, as a proportion of these patients will become hypoglycemic again after treatment.

Severe hypoglycemia

- Patients should carry a card or wear a bracelet or necklace identifying themselves as diabetic, and these should be looked for in unconscious patients. The diagnosis of severe hypoglycemia resulting in confusion or coma is simple and can usually be made on clinical grounds, backed by an 'on the spot' finger-stick blood test.
  - ◇ If real doubt exists, blood should be taken for glucose estimation before treatment is given, as long as this does not delay treatment for more than a short period (i.e. 1–2 minutes).
- Unconscious patients should be given either intramuscular glucagon (1 mg) or intravenous glucose (25–50 ml of 50% dextrose solution) followed by a flush of normal saline to preserve the vein (since 50% dextrose scleroses veins).
  - ◇ Glucagon acts by mobilizing hepatic glycogen, and works almost as rapidly as glucose. It is simple to administer and can be given at home by relatives. It does not work after a prolonged fast.

Insulin treatment

◆ As with milder hypoglycemia, oral administration of slowly absorbed carbohydrate, once the patient is more alert and able to comply, and continuing careful observation for several hours are important, so that recurrence of hypoglycemia can be prevented or promptly recognized and dealt with.

Preventing hypoglycemia

◆ If a pattern of hypoglycemic episodes is evident, then hypoglycemic agents such as sulfonylureas and insulin should be adjusted accordingly.

◆ Patients on insulin, especially basal–bolus insulin, can be taught how to adjust insulin doses temporarily while waiting to see their treating physician. Ideally, patients would have been taught, and would have understood, that the insulin dose to be lowered is the dose preceding the hypoglycemic events:

◇ If a patient frequently has hypoglycemic events mid-morning, it is the rapid-acting insulin at breakfast that has to be decreased.

◇ If the patient has hypoglycemic events upon awakening in the morning, then it is the long-acting insulin dose that has to be reduced.

◆ Often, patients who do not recognize that the insulin dose has to be reduced consume extra carbohydrates to prevent low blood glucose.

Other complications or adverse effects from insulin treatment

◆ Hypoglycemia is the most common complication of treatment with insulin or insulin secretagogues, but there are other considerations (**195**).

◆ Weight gain occurs with insulin treatment, since insulin has anabolic effects. Weight gain can also result from hypoglycemic episodes, as patients overcompensate by eating more calories than needed. It is, therefore, especially important to counsel patients on an appropriate diet.

◆ True insulin allergy is rare; allergy is more often due to the additives in the insulin preparations. For true insulin allergy, desensitization can be performed by allergy specialists.

◇ Anti-insulin antibodies can develop in response to exogenous insulin, but generally do not affect the therapeutic effect of insulin.

◆ Lipoatrophy and lipohypertrophy may occur at insulin injection sites used repeatedly (**196**). Management includes avoiding those sites until improvement is seen, and rotating injection sites to avoid these local reactions.

◆ Edema can occur, and may be more frequent when insulin is used in combination with TZDs.

Rotate injection sites to avoid local reactions.

Complications of insulin treatment

Allergy
Local or general

Dose-dependent
Hypoglycemia
Weight gain (due to the anabolic action of insulin)

Not dose-dependent
Lipohypertrophy (due to repeated injections at the same site)
Lipoatrophy (rare now with purified insulin)
Insulin edema (especially just after the start of treatment)

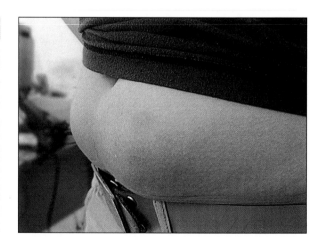

195 Complications of treatment. Side-effects of insulin treatment, such as allergic reaction, are rare, but they do occur in some patients.

196 Lipohypertrophy at insulin injection sites. Lipohypertrophy may lead to poor glycemic control, as insulin absorption can be significantly delayed.

Insulin treatment

CHAPTER 15

Special management considerations

The diabetic inpatient

◆ Diabetes is a chronic illness, mostly managed in the outpatient setting. When a diabetic patient is admitted to the hospital for reasons other than diabetes, the focus of treatment is the illness triggering the admission.

◆ Diabetic patients who have poor control before admission may continue to have poor control in the hospital. Patients who lack dietary discipline may experience unexpected hypoglycemia and a decrease in insulin requirements with imposed dietary compliance caused by hospitalization.

◆ Patients who were in good control before admission now find themselves with elevated blood glucoses since they are sick, and the dosing of their insulin is left to physicians who may not pay careful attention to their glycemic control.

◆ The risk of mortality and complications increases as the level of hyperglycemia increases (**197**).
   ◇ Mortality is higher in hyperglycemic versus nonhyperglycemic patients.
   ◇ Mortality in those without a previous diagnosis of diabetes (i.e. patients who have new hyperglycemia) has been shown to be even greater in a few studies – either because hyperglycemia is a marker for worse prognosis or because newly diagnosed diabetes was frequently left untreated (**198**). In support of the latter, patients known to have diabetes have improved outcomes when aggressively managed with insulin.

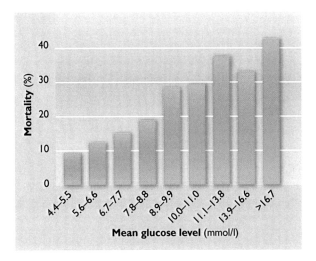

197 Hyperglycemia in critically ill patients. Hyperglycemia is associated with a significantly increased risk of mortality. *Adapted from Krinsley JS, 2003.*

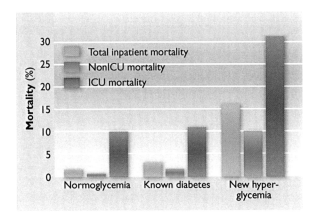

198 Inpatient mortality. Patients with new hyperglycemia admitted to both critical care areas and general wards had a significantly higher mortality rate than patients with a known history of diabetes or normoglycemia. *Adapted from Umpierrez GE et al, 2002.*

- In the critically ill, the use of insulin infusion protocols in the intensive care unit has facilitated the control of hyperglycemia.
- Morbidity and mortality are lower in intensively treated patients achieving excellent glucose control.
  - ◇ In one study of hyperglycemic patients admitted to the surgical intensive care unit, the use of an insulin infusion protocol to achieve blood glucose levels of <6.0 mmol/l (108 mg/dl) was associated with significantly less mortality and less incidence of complications (such as acute renal failure, critical care neuropathy, septicemia, and the need for blood transfusions) compared to conventional treatment. Of note, only 13% of these patients had a known history of diabetes.
  - ◇ The same study was performed in the medical intensive care unit; in this group, intensive insulin infusion reduced morbidity but not mortality.
  - ◇ In cardiothoracic surgery, the use of insulin infusion protocols in diabetic patients immediately following coronary artery bypass graft resulted in a reduced incidence of deep sternal wound infection, and thus a decreased length of hospital stay.
- Recent studies in critically ill patients suggest, however, that a tight glucose target of 4.4–6.1 mmol/l (80–110 mg/dl) may have to be re-evaluated. Studies such as the VISEP and NICE-SUGAR show either no benefit, or a greater risk of hypoglycemia and mortality, with tighter control.
- Insulin infusions are broadly recommended for perioperative care and details of such management are to be found in more specialized sources.
- In the noncritically ill patient on the regular hospital ward, the ongoing use of retroactive sliding scale insulin therapy, despite recommendations to the contrary, is one of the reasons why hyperglycemia is perpetuated.
- The use of basal insulin (in the form of NPH [isophane] insulin, detemir insulin or glargine insulin) and, if necessary, prandial insulin, can prevent hyperglycemia, whereas sliding scales are reactive and only treat patients when the blood glucoses are high.

- Detemir or glargine 10 IU daily for insulin-naïve patients, or 0.15 IU/kg daily for patients with features of insulin resistance, is a typical starting dose to provide patients with basal insulin in the hospital. However, many acutely ill patients will require doses of 0.3 IU/kg or higher.
- Insulin pumps present a unique problem: patients with these are usually independent and attuned to their insulin needs. However, if they are too ill to manipulate their pumps and calculate insulin doses, it may be better to put these patients on basal and prandial subcutaneous insulin if the hospital staff cannot operate the pump. This decision can be arrived at based on the patient's clinical state and the individual hospital's policy, if any exists, regarding allowing the patient to self-administer insulin.

Diabetes and surgery

- It is now accepted, and supported by clinical trial results, that efforts to achieve near-normal glycemia during and after major surgery, particularly cardiothoracic surgery, and in surgical intensive care patients, will significantly decrease mortality and postoperative infection, and may also decrease the need for transfusion, need for dialysis, and critical care neuropathy (**199**).
- When an emergency major surgical procedure is required in a diabetic patient it is, therefore, mandatory to institute immediately an insulin infusion regimen that aims to achieve and sustain near normal glucose levels (4–8 mmol/l [72–144 mg/dl]) (**200**).
  - ◇ Relevant medical, nursing, and intensive care staff should be trained in the use of an algorithm-based insulin infusion regimen (**201**).
- Experienced medical and nursing staff may assume that hypoglycemia is the major risk to the severely ill postoperative patient, but the adverse consequences of hyperglycemia probably outweigh the minor risks posed by hypoglycemia in such patients.

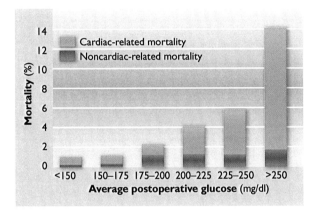

199 Intensive insulin therapy in critically ill patients. In a study of 1548 patients, intensive therapy reduced both ICU and general in-hospital mortality. *Adapted from van den Berghe G, et al, 2001.*

200 Coronary artery bypass graft surgery and hyperglycemia. There is a clear relationship between high glucose levels and high in-hospital cardiac-related mortality. *Adapted from Furnary AP, Gao G, et al. 2003.*

Insulin-treated diabetes regimen

Stop long-acting and/or intermediate insulin the day before surgery, substitute short-acting insulin, and start insulin infusion

Use intravenous 10% dextrose (500 ml infused at 100 ml/h) and soluble (regular in US) insulin (1–3 IU/h) perioperatively with potassium chloride (10 mmol [10 mEq] in 500 ml)

Postoperatively, the infusion is maintained until the patient is able to eat. Other fluids must be given through a separate intravenous line

Monitor glucose and potassium levels and adjust amounts in infusion while keeping the rate constant

When transitioning patient from infusion to subcutaneous insulin the first injection of basal insulin should be administered at least 2 h before the infusion is discontinued

201 Insulin therapy for hospitalized patients. Staff should be trained in administration of an insulin infusion.

Major surgery

◆ For major surgery that is elective, rather than emergency, efforts should be made to optimize glycemic control and electrolytes before admission to hospital (**202**).
  ◇ If that seems unlikely to be achieved on an outpatient basis, consider admitting the patient a day early for intensive insulin management preoperatively.
◆ Tight glycemic control postoperatively should be just as outlined for emergency surgery.
◆ These principles should apply equally to type 1 and type 2 diabetes.

202 Elective surgery. Plan to optimize glycemic control.

Diabetes management for surgery

Management is by a team; liaison between the diabetes team and the anesthetist is ideal

Metabolic control should be optimized before the operation. For emergency surgery, metabolic disturbances should be carefully managed

Use insulin therapy when in doubt

Put the patient at the beginning of the list at the start of the day, if practicable

Electrolyte disturbances should be corrected before surgery, when feasible

Special management considerations

Diet- or tablet-treated diabetes

Omit short-acting agents (e.g. sulfonylureas) on the morning of the operation
Omit long-acting sulfonylureas (e.g. glibenclamide/glyburide) at least 24 h before nonemergency surgery, and manage glycemia with insulin
Avoid glucose- and lactate-containing fluids in minor operations when possible
Avoid metformin perioperatively and if radiological contrast is required
For all major operations consider need for insulin treatment. For relatively minor procedures it may be sufficient simply to omit oral agents on the morning of surgery, and resume when the patient starts eating again

203 Hospitalized patients and oral therapy. Oral anti-hyperglycemic therapy should be discontinued and insulin therapy initiated if needed.

◆ Where the patient's usual treatment is with oral agents these should be discontinued at least 24 hours before surgery, and insulin instituted (**203**).

◆ Ideally, the operation should be scheduled at the start of the operating list, if practicable.

Minor surgery
◆ For minor surgery there can be a more individualized approach, with some basic ground rules:
  ◇ Insulin secretagogues, especially the longer acting, should be discontinued at least 24 hours before surgery.
  ◇ If use of contrast material in imaging peri- or postoperatively is anticipated, metformin should be discontinued the day before.
◆ Insulin glargine or detemir, given the evening before surgery, may be an alternative to insulin infusion, but published data are lacking.
◆ For short and very simple procedures it may be sufficient to omit oral agents or short-acting insulin on the morning of surgery.

Surgery and blood pressure
◆ As a general medical consideration it is accepted that control of blood pressure should be achieved before elective surgery.

Conception, contraception, and pregnancy

◆ Diabetes, both type 1 and type 2, confers a greater maternal and fetal risk than in women without diabetes. Diabetes management extends to all periods of pregnancy and includes the pre-pregnancy planning period and the postnatal phase (**204**, **205**).

◆ Modern management of pregnancy in diabetic women means that outcomes in specialized centers approach those in nondiabetic pregnancy.
  ◇ Before the discovery of insulin in 1921, most women with type 1 diabetes did not survive to reproductive age; the few pregnancies reported suffered a 50% perinatal and maternal mortality rate. Even 50 years ago both the maternal and neonatal morbidity and mortality were substantial.
  ◇ The subsequent transformation was due to meticulous metabolic control throughout the three trimesters of pregnancy and general improvements in medical and obstetric management (**206**).

◆ Glycemic control at the time of conception and in the early weeks of pregnancy is particularly important, as maternal hyperglycemia and/or accompanying metabolic disturbance during organogenesis increase the risk of congenital malformation in the fetus.

◆ However, even with good glycemic control and improved obstetric services, rates of congenital malformation and perinatal death associated with pregnancy in type 1 diabetes continue to exceed those in nondiabetic women (**207**).
  ◇ Whether this is because not all diabetic women receive obstetric care in specialized centers is a matter of conjecture, and while a case can be made for such a policy, its implementation would be difficult to enforce in most healthcare systems.

Diabetes management should cover the prepregnancy planning period.

Management points for diabetes in pregnancy

Pre-pregnancy counseling to optimize blood glucose control and thereby limit risk of congenital malformations

Optimize blood glucose control with 1 h postprandial blood glucose between 4 and 8 mmol/l (72–144 mg/dl) and HbA1c (or fructosamine) in the normal range

Monitor blood glucose control. Ketoacidosis in pregnancy carries a 50% fetal mortality, but maternal hypoglycemia is relatively well tolerated by the fetus

Limit calorie intake in obesity (30% decrease) and avoid refined carbohydrate

Insulin therapy if blood glucose does not achieve targets. Use multiple injections or insulin subcutaneous pump, as insulin requirement rises progressively during the 2nd trimester, levelling off thereafter

Avoid oral hypoglycemic agents unless strong indication

Review in joint diabetes/antenatal clinic at intervals of ≤2 weeks. The aim should be outpatient management with a spontaneous vaginal delivery at term. Retinopathy and nephropathy may deteriorate. Expert fundoscopy and urine testing for protein undertaken at booking, at 28 weeks, and before delivery

Delivery should be in hospital. Obstetric problems include stillbirth, fetopelvic disproportion, hydramnios, and pre-eclampsia. Assess pregnancy staging using ultrasound. Cesarean section is often required

Management plan for diabetes in the three trimesters

FIRST TRIMESTER

Mother	Folate supplements (to reduce congenital malformation risk)
	Stop smoking; avoid alcohol, ACEIs, statins
	Optimize glycemic control
	Screen for diabetes complications
Baby	Ultrasound scan (for congenital anomalies)

SECOND TRIMESTER

Mother	Stop smoking, avoid alcohol
	Optimize glycemic control (insulin dose increases)
	Screen and treat diabetes complications
	Monitor and treat blood pressure
Baby	Ultrasound scan (for congenital anomalies, growth)

THIRD TRIMESTER

Mother	Stop smoking, avoid alcohol, check drugs
	Optimize glycemic control (insulin dose increases to 34–36 weeks)
	Screen and treat diabetes complications
	Monitor and treat blood pressure
	Check for pre-eclampsia (twice as common as normal)
Baby	Ultrasound scan (for congenital anomalies, growth)
	Plan delivery

204 Management points. Optimization of blood glucose is key to successful management.

205 Management plan. Management of early pregnancy is important to reduce the risk of congenital anomalies.

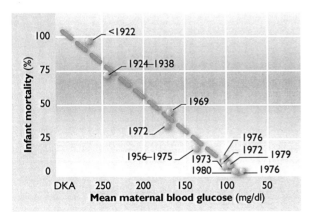

206 Infant mortality. A review of the major studies over the last century revealed that as maternal blood glucose concentrations decreased, infant mortality also decreased. *Adapted from Jovanovic and Peterson.*

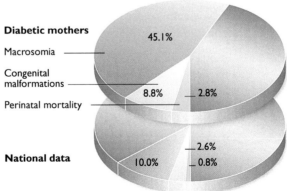

207 Perinatal outcomes. Women with type 1 diabetes in the Netherlands in 1999–2000 showed a 3–4-fold greater risk of obstetric complications compared to national data. *Adapted from Evers IM, de Valk HW, et al. 2004.*

Contraception and diabetes

◆ Because the issue of periconceptual glycemic control is so important, pregnancy in diabetes should preferably be planned, therefore contraception is an important part of management.

◆ There may sometimes be situations related to diabetes in which it is better to advise against pregnancy altogether, though that decision is ultimately for the patient to make (see p. 182).

◆ The options for contraception are as for non-diabetic individuals, and an individual approach should be taken to deciding which is appropriate for the particular patient. Methods other than the contraceptive pill, tubal ligation, and vasectomy have significant 'failure' rates – perhaps as high as 4–5% for IUCD and condom, rising to at least 20% for the rhythm method.

◆ Regarding the contraceptive pill, the only *specific* point of relevance in diabetes relates to the metabolic effects associated with estrogen.

  ◇ High-dose estrogen combined pills may cause an increase in glycemia, necessitating an increase in insulin dosage; this is not the case with low-dose estrogen pills, which are prescribed much more.

  ◇ Lipid levels are less likely to be perturbed by low-dose than high-dose combined pills.

  ◇ In women with clinical macrovascular disease or with other significant risk factors such as strong family history, smoking, hypertension, or hyperlipidemia, the use of combined estrogen–progesterone contraception needs to be carefully considered, as would be the case in women without diabetes. An increased risk of thromboembolic disease accompanies use of a combined oral contraceptive pill, though it is less with low-dose formulations.

◆ Progestogen-only pills are not associated with metabolic or lipid disturbance, and therefore may be considered particularly suitable for women with diabetes. They can lead to menstrual irregularity such as intermenstrual bleeding, or sometimes amenorrhea.

  ◇ Intermenstrual bleeding may be resolved by increasing the dose temporarily for just a few cycles.

  ◇ Once it has been established that the onset of amenorrhea is associated with a negative pregnancy test the patient can be reassured that the amenorrhea is a natural effect of the progestogen inhibiting ovulation.

Glucose monitoring and glycemic goals in pregnancy

◆ The optimal method of glucose monitoring in pregnancy has been reasonably well, indeed uniquely, studied.

  ◇ Most studies of the utility of glucose monitoring in insulin-treated diabetes apart from pregnancy have concentrated on preprandial and fasting glucose.

  ◇ However, a study of preprandial glucose monitoring in women with insulin-treated gestational diabetes suggested that this strategy did not adequately reflect strict glycemic control or decrease the risk of macrosomia.

  ◇ A subsequent randomized study in a similar cohort showed that, in comparison to preprandial monitoring, postprandial testing led to a greater decrease in HbA1c, lower mean infant birth weight with fewer 'weight-related' complications such as cephalopelvic disproportion, and less likelihood of cesarean section and neonatal hypoglycemia. However, this study has been criticized on the grounds that the preprandial glucose target was set at a relatively high level (3.3–5.9 mmol/l [60–106 mg/dl]) whereas the postprandial target was relatively low (7.8 mmol/l [140 mg/dl]).

High-dose estrogen combined contraceptive pills may cause an increase in glycemia.

Obstetric outcome in relation to pre- and postprandial blood glucose monitoring

VARIABLE	PREPRANDIAL (n = 31)	POSTPRANDIAL (n = 30)
Delivery gestational age (wks)	36.9 (1.5)	36.7 (2.5)
Weight gain (kg)	15.0 (5.2)	15.9 (6.5)
Insulin dose Prepregnancy Units/day Units/kg Change	50.0 (23.2) 105.0 (51.3) 1.2 (0.5) 50.2 (35.7)	51.3 (25.1) 120.4 (32.3) 1.4 (0.5) 65 (49.0)
Cesarean section Total For suspected disproportion	21/31 (68%) 8/31 (26%)	14/30 (47%) 7/30 (23%)
Pre-eclampsia	6/28 (21%)	1/30 (3%)
Mean glycated hemoglobin (%) [mmol/mol] Initial Final	7.6 [59] 6.3 [46]	7.4 [56] 6.0 [42]
Mean capillary glucose (mmol/l) [mg/dl] Trimester 2 (before breakfast) Trimester 3 (before breakfast)	7.7 [138.6] (1.8) 7.0 [126.0] (1.3)	7.0 [126.0] (2.0) 7.0 [126.0] (2.0)
Fructosamine (μmol/l) Trimester 2 Trimester 3	250.4 (37.6) 214.4 (27.2)	240.3 (33.2) 213.4 (32.8)
Success in glycemic control (%) Trimester 2 Trimester 3	29.4 (11) 30.3 (11)	51.6 (19) 55.5 (20)

Data presented as mean (SD) or number (%) where appropriate.
Adapted, with permission, from Manderson JG, Patterson CC, Hadden DR, et al. 2003.

◇ A randomized study with glucose targets identical to those in the above study, but carried out in type 1 diabetic women from 16 weeks' gestation, showed that postprandial monitoring, as compared with preprandial, was associated with greater success in achieving glycemic targets in the second and third trimesters and significantly less likelihood of pre-eclampsia (**208**).

◆ There is now a consensus that in pregnancy the aim should be to achieve glucose levels of less than 7.8 mmol/l (140 mg/dl) 1 hour after meals. There is more debate about appropriate preprandial targets, with some investigators suggesting a target of 3.3–4.4 mmol/l (60–80 mg/dl) rather than the more conservative one of <5.9 mmol/l (106 mg/dl).

208 Glucose monitoring. In this study, 61 women with type 1 diabetes were randomly assigned at 16 weeks' gestation to preprandial or postprandial blood glucose monitoring throughout pregnancy. Maternal age, parity, age of onset of diabetes, number of previous miscarriages, smoking status, social class, weight gain in pregnancy, and compliance with therapy were similar in both groups. The postprandial monitoring group had a significantly reduced incidence of pre-eclampsia and greater success in achieving glycemic targets.

In pregnancy, the aim should be to achieve postprandial glucose levels of less than 7.8 mmol/l.

Special management considerations

Type 1 diabetes patients

◆ Prepregnancy counseling, with efforts to achieve near normal glycemia, and the planned introduction of folate 5 mg, should ideally be the rule at an early stage in adult life.

◆ Inevitably, many women become pregnant when HbA1c is still elevated.

◆ An appreciation of the effect of pregnancy on insulin needs is crucial.

◆ During the first trimester insulin requirements are fairly stable, though the actual diagnosis of pregnancy will often lead to a change in the level of self-care, and if dietary habits alter (i.e. calorie intake decreases) there may be a need for adjusting the insulin dosage downwards. On the other hand, in those women with elevated HbA1c an alteration in the insulin dose (usually an increase) will be required to optimize glycemic control rapidly.
  ◇ Patients not already on an intensive insulin regimen of multiple injections or a subcutaneous insulin infusion pump should be strongly advised to adopt one or the other.

◆ In the second trimester, insulin needs rise steadily, often to more than double the pre-pregnancy dose, and then tend to level off or occasionally even fall slightly in the final few weeks (**209**).
  ◇ The precise cause of the increasing insulin need is not known, but is probably related to the rise in hormones like cortisol, progesterone, and human placental lactogen.

◆ Management of glycemia during labor is best achieved by intravenous infusion of insulin and glucose, the aim being to maintain normal glucose levels.

◆ Immediately postpartum the insulin resistance of pregnancy decreases, so the insulin dose may decrease to low levels, even zero, for a few days; thereafter, insulin should be resumed at a dosage appropriate for prepregnancy needs.

An appreciation of the effect of pregnancy on insulin needs is crucial.

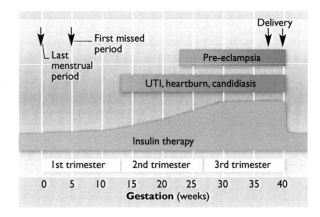

209 **Impact of diabetes on the mother.** Insulin needs rise rapidly in the second trimester.

◆ In the sense that insulin therapy is a necessity for women with type 1 diabetes, its 'safety' in pregnancy has been established through common usage; the outcome for both the mother and the fetus would be clearly disastrous in the absence of insulin therapy.

◆ Insulin analogs, prescribed increasingly along with or in preference to human insulin in non-pregnant diabetic patients, have not been specifically tested for safety in human pregnancy. Inevitably, therefore, the package inserts of analog insulins caution against the lack of safety data as to their use in pregnancy.
  ◇ With each new analog, concerns are raised about potential for harm, for example through affinity for placental receptors of insulin-like growth factors. However, to date, the lack of evidence for adverse effects supports the emerging view that insulin analogs are probably just as safe as human and animal insulin.
  ◇ It is unlikely that the safety issue will ever be strictly tested in randomized controlled trials in pregnancy, and probably true that the majority of diabetologists with wide experience in pregnancy treatment would regard current insulin analogs as safe for use.
  ◇ Each woman and her partner need to make an informed choice between the lack of evidence of an adverse effect of insulin analogs, the known risk of diabetic pregnancy, and the risk of poor diabetes control versus the potential benefit of good glucose control using insulin analogs.

Type 2 diabetes patients

◆ The rising prevalence of type 2 diabetes in women of childbearing age has resulted in increasing numbers of pregnant women with pre-existing diabetes.

◆ Unless stringent glycemic control is readily achieved through dietary management the consensus is that insulin treatment is appropriate.

◇ Initial insulin needs are likely to be greater than in type 1 diabetes because of the pre-existing insulin resistance associated with type 2 diabetes, but the principles of treatment are essentially the same.

◆ Many diabetic women, on learning that they are pregnant, make a renewed effort with dietary care and their general well-being. So, in theory at least, since glycemia in type 2 diabetes is potentially more responsive to lifestyle change than in type 1 diabetes, insulin requirements may be individually more variable.

◆ It is likely that some women with type 2 diabetes could maintain satisfactory control with oral agents, but studies of this are limited.

◇ At present the use of oral agents is not acknowledged as the 'standard of care', though many patients with diabetes and polycystic ovary syndrome are becoming pregnant whilst on metformin, and results to date suggest that the drug has no adverse effect on the fetus.

◆ A retrospective survey in South Africa found that, despite the achievement of comparable glycemic control when glibenclamide and metformin were used rather than insulin, there were higher perinatal mortality and stillbirth rates (**210**), but such adverse effects from these oral agents have not been confimed in other studies.

210 Oral glucose-lowering agents in pregnancy.
In an analysis of 379 women with type 2 diabetes using oral hypoglycemic agents (metformin and glibenclamide) subdivided into three groups according to therapy, increased perinatal mortality was associated with the use of sulfonylureas or sulfonylureas plus metformin. Conversion from oral agents to insulin was protective for perinatal mortality compared with oral agents alone.

Comparison of insulin and oral glucose-lowering agents in pregnancy

	ORAL AGENTS ALONE	ORAL AGENTS → INSULIN	DIET/INSULIN
Birth weight (g)	3185.2 ± 103.3 (n = 90)	3259.0 ± 52.3 (n = 244)	3238.8 ± 140.5 (n = 29)
No. of outcomes/ no. of pregnancies			
Perinatal mortality	11/88 (12.5%)	7/248 (2.8%)	1/30 (3.3%)
Stillbirth rate	8/88 (9.1%)	5/248 (2.0%)	1/30 (3.3%)
Neonatal death rate	3/87 (3.4%)	2/248 (0.8%)	0/30 (0.0%)
No. of outcomes/ no of pregnancies			
Fetal anomaly	5/88 (5.7%)	5/248 (2.0%)	0/30 (0.0%)
Cesarean section	55/88 (62.5%)	146/244 (59.8%)	18/31 (58.1%)
Neonatal hypoglycemia	18/75 (24%)	37/196 (18.9%)	5/22 (22.7%)
Macrosomia	21/90 (23.3%)	44/245 (18%)	5/29 (17.2%)
Pre-eclampsia	3/87 (3.4%)	5/239 (2.1%)	0/33 (0.0%)
Neonatal jaundice	14/75 (18.7%)	21/199 (10.6%)	2/22 (9.1%)

Adapted, with permission, from Ekpebegh CO, Coetzee EJ, van der Merwe L, et al 2007.

Special management considerations

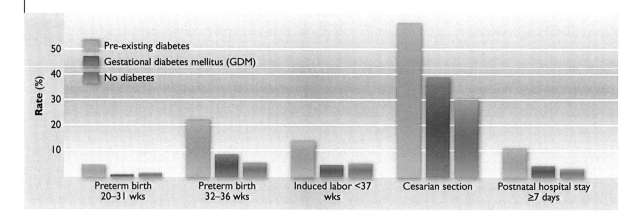

211 Pregnancy outcomes. The Australian Institute of Health and Welfare analysis of National Perinatal Data Collection data found that mothers with pre-existing diabetes have higher rates of adverse pregnancy outcomes than mothers without diabetes or with GDM.

Risks to the diabetic mother

- Theoretically the risk of maternal mortality is higher in the diabetic than nondiabetic pregnancy (**211**, **212**). This relates to:
  - ◇ Risk of ketoacidosis if appropriate attention is not paid to glycemic control.
  - ◇ Increased labor risks if there is fetal macrosomia.
  - ◇ Increased risk of cardiac or renal failure in the presence of established advanced microvascular or macrovascular disease.
  - ◇ Increased risk of pre-eclampsia.

Risks of diabetic pregnancy

MATERNAL RISKS

Metabolic deterioration

Microvascular complications progress

Macrovascular complications

Risk of urinary tract infection increased

Risk of pre-eclampsia increased

Rates of cesarean section increased

FETAL RISKS

Risk of congenital malformations increased (cardiac, sacral agenesis, spina bifida)

Rates of stillbirth increased

Perinatal morbidity and mortality increased

Neonatal complications increased (fetal distress, jaundice, hypoglycemia)

Risk of diabetes in later life increased

- It is important to screen all pregnant diabetic women for the presence of microvascular complications as soon as pregnancy is diagnosed.
- The pre-existence of complications is not necessarily a reason to advise against pregnancy, but women with diabetes should be made aware that microvascular complications can worsen suddenly and considerably during pregnancy despite improving glycemic control. Reasons for strongly advising against pregnancy include:
  - ◇ Clinical ischemic heart disease holds greatly increased maternal risk of mortality, and, arguably with the increasing prevalence of type 2 diabetes in younger patients, we may expect to see more patients in that situation.
  - ◇ Advanced nephropathy, particularly with severe hypertension or proteinuria, is associated with greatly increased risk to both mother and fetus.
  - ◇ Active proliferative retinopathy.
  - ◇ Severe symptomatic autonomic neuropathy.

Microvascular complications can worsen considerably during pregnancy, despite improving glycemic control.

---

212 Pregnancy risks. Diabetes during pregnancy significantly increases the risks to both mother and child.

Gestational diabetes mellitus (GDM)

◆ GDM occurs when abnormal glucose tolerance develops during pregnancy in a woman not known to have diabetes before pregnancy, unless she has had GDM in a previous pregnancy.

◆ Usually the abnormal glucose tolerance resolves after delivery, but women with GDM are quite likely to develop it again in a subsequent pregnancy, and are at considerably increased risk of developing type 2 diabetes in the future.

◇ Progression to diabetes is around 30% over 7–10 years, or in some particularly suscepti-ble populations as high as 50% in 5 years, suggesting that GDM is a 'prediabetic' state.

◇ Women who are obese, older, have first-degree relatives with diabetes, have a previous history of poor pregnancy outcome, have a history of large-for-gestational-age babies, or belong to an ethnic/racial group with a known high prevalence of type 2 diabetes are particularly at risk for GDM.

◆ About 2% of pregnant white Europeans develop gestational diabetes. A small percentage of cases have diabetes-associated antibodies and progress to type 1 diabetes mellitus.

◆ *Screening.* All women over age 25 and with BMI above normal should be assessed for diabetes early in pregnancy, unless they have absolutely none of the risk factors mentioned above. If they are found not to have GDM they should be tested again between 24 and 28 weeks and more fre-quently if at particularly high risk.

◆ GDM is usually asymptomatic.

◆ Diagnostic criteria have been established for GDM (**213**). The definition is based on either a 3-hour/100-g (ADA, 2001) or a 2-hour/75-g (WHO, 1999) oral glucose tolerance test (OGTT). These criteria are still a matter for debate, though there is a general move towards standardization.

◇ The International Association of the Diabetes and Pregnancy Study Groups (IADPSG) fetal outcome-based definition, using 2-hour 75 g OGTT data from the worldwide Hyper-glycemia and Adverse Pregnancy Outcome (HAPO) study, is being adopted in many countries.

◆ IADPSG has also published a strategy to detect unrecognized type 2 diabetes at the first prenatal visit, so that therapy can be started immediately.

Diagnostic criteria for GDM

Plasma glucose (mmol/l [mg/dl])	IADPSG	WHO	ADA
Fasting	5.1 [92]	7.0 [126]	5.3 [95]
1 h	10.0 [180]	–	10.0 [180]
2 h	8.5 [153]	7.8 [140]	8.6 [155]
3 h*	–	–	7.8 [140]

* 100-g load only

213 Diagnostic criteria. The definition of GDM is based on an oral glucose tolerance test (OGTT). The IADPSG threshold values of venous plasma glucose (one or more to be equalled or exceeded) are listed, as well as previous systems from the WHO and ADA, which are still used in some centers.

◆ Initial treatment for GDM is with diet, though there is no consensus as to which one is best. There have been no randomized trials addressing this issue and there are no data, other than a possible reduction in the risk of macrosomia, to support any particular intervention.

◆ Insulin treatment, required in about 30% of cases, is initiated if postprandial glucose cannot be maintained at less than 7.8 mmol/l (140 mg/dl) with diet.

◇ Insulin does not cross the placenta.

◆ Oral agents such as metformin and second-generation sulfonylureas may be of value when the hyperglycemia is just above target levels, though caution should be exercised, and these agents remain the second line of treatment.

◆ GDM is associated with the obstetric and neonatal problems described for pre-existing diabetes, except that there is no increase in the rate of con-genital abnormalities. The later onset of glucose intolerance in gestational diabetes means that such abnormalities – a result of glucose intoler-ance in the first trimester – do not occur.

◆ Hospital admission may be required if the patient is symptomatic, has ketonuria or a marked hyper-glycemia (>15 mmol/l, 270 mg/dl).

Fetal macrosomia is the major risk, affecting up to 40%. This in turn increases the risk of birth injuries due to the large size of the fetus, but earlier delivery to avoid birth injuries inevitably increases the risks associated with prematurity.

◇ Keeping the postprandial glucose below 7.8 mmol/l (140 mg/dl) has been shown to reduce the likelihood of macrosomia and its attendant risks, though it does not completely normalize the risk.

The occurrence of GDM must be regarded as an indication for preventive measures postpartum against the development of type 2 diabetes in the future.

◇ All such women should be encouraged to continue lifestyle measures (diet and exercise) after pregnancy even if glucose levels have returned to normal.

◇ Interest in the possible role of TZD treatment in the prevention of type 2 diabetes in this population (see p. 147) is now limited due to safety concerns.

Labor and delivery

Labor and delivery are potentially hazardous for the diabetic mother and her baby. The need for cesarean section – used more commonly in diabetes – should be frequently reviewed; the aim should be for natural childbirth as near to term as possible.

Indications for elective delivery by the abdomen include:

◇ Malpresentation.
◇ Disproportion between child and birth canal.
◇ Intrauterine growth retardation.
◇ Fetal distress.
◇ Pre-eclampsia.

Insulin requirements are low during labor and insulin can be given by continuous intravenous insulin infusion (typically 2–4 IU/h of fast-acting soluble insulin) plus 10% glucose infusion at 125 ml/h (i.e. 1 l every 8 h) with regular blood glucose (usually capillary sample) monitoring.

After delivery the insulin requirements fall to pre-pregnancy levels and the insulin infusion rate should be reduced by half initially.

Neonatal problems

Neonatal hypoglycemia may occur in infants born to a diabetic mother.

The mechanism of neonatal hypoglycemia is as follows:

◇ Maternal glucose crosses the placenta, but insulin does not.
◇ The fetal islets hypersecrete to combat maternal hyperglycemia.
◇ The neonatal glucose falls to hypoglycemic levels when the umbilical cord is severed.

Other problems in neonates include:

◇ Respiratory distress syndrome or hyaline membrane disease (a disease of the lung membrane that causes respiratory difficulty; uncommon now).
◇ Transient hypertrophic cardiomyopathy (30% affected on ultrasound).
◇ Hypocalcemia (50%) and hypomagnesemia (80%).
◇ Polycythemia (12%) and jaundice (60%).

Maternal diabetes, especially when poorly controlled, is associated with fetal macrosomia (defined as large-for-gestational dates) (**214**) and accelerated fetal growth (**215**).

214 **Macrosomia.** Macrosomia in an infant of a mother with diabetes (left), compared with a normal-sized infant of a non-diabetic mother (right). *Photo courtesy Dr Anne Dornhorst.*

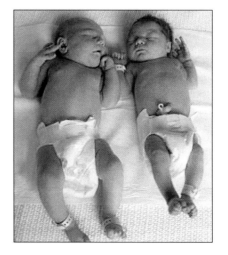

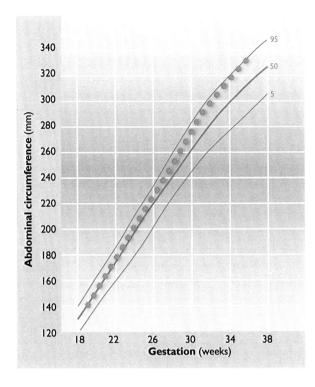

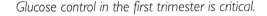

215 Accelerated fetal growth. Abdominal circumference in the fetus of a mother with type 2 diabetes.

216 Congenital malformations. Diabetes is associated with an increased risk of major and minor fetal abnormality.

Common major congenital malformations	
Cardiac	Great vessel anomalies Septal defects
Central nervous system	Anencephaly Spina bifida
Skeletal and facial	Caudal regression syndrome Cleft palate or lip Arthrogryposis
Genitourinary tract	Renal agenesis Ureteric duplication

◆ The infant of a diabetic mother is more susceptible to congenital malformations and also to hyaline membrane disease than infants of similar maturity of nondiabetic mothers (**216**, **217**).

 ◇ These abnormalities are principally related to hyperglycemia, congenital malformations being largely determined by hyperglycemia in the first trimester – the critical period with regard to organogenesis (**218**).

 ◇ When a pregnancy is planned, optimal metabolic control should be sought before conception.

Glucose control in the first trimester is critical.

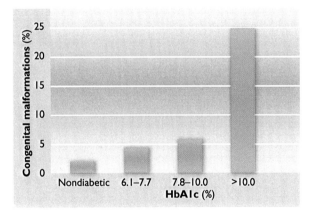

217 Malformation risk. The risk of congenital malformations in newborns of women with type 1 diabetes is about twice as high as in the general population, even when HbA1c is normal. The risk increases sharply with poor blood glucose control. *Adapted from Taylor and Davison, 2007.*

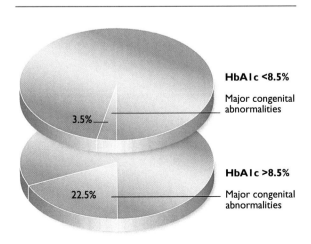

HbA1c <8.5%

Major congenital abnormalities

3.5%

HbA1c >8.5%

Major congenital abnormalities

22.5%

218 First-trimester hyperglycemia. HbA1c above 8.5% in early pregnancy is associated with an almost seven-fold increase in major congenital abnormalities.

Alwan N, Tuffnell DJ, West J (2009) Treatments for gestational diabetes. *Cochrane Database Syst Rev.* Jul 8;(3):CD003395.

American Diabetes Association (2008) Economic costs of diabetes in the U.S. in 2007. *Diabetes Care* 31:596–615.

American Diabetes Association (2012) Standards of Medical Care in Diabetes–2012. *Diabetes Care* 35:S11–S63.

Astrup A, Rössner S, Van Gaal L, Rissanen A, Niskanen L, Al Hakim M, Madsen J, Rasmussen MF, Lean ME; NN8022–1807 Study Group (2009) Effects of liraglutide in the treatment of obesity: a randomised, double-blind, placebo-controlled study. *Lancet* 374:1606–1616.

BARI Investigators (2007) The final 10-year follow-up results from the BARI randomized trial. *J Am Coll Cardiol* 49:1600–1606.

Bhatt DL, Marso SP, Lincoff AM, Wolski KE, Ellis SG, Topol EJ (2000) Abciximab reduces mortality in diabetics following percutaneous coronary inter-vention. *J Am Coll Cardiol* 35:922–928.

Black HR, Davis B, Barzilay J, Nwachuku C, Baimbridge C, Marginean H, Wright JT Jr, Basile J, Wong ND, Whelton P, Dart RA, Thadani U (2008) Antihypertensive and Lipid-Lowering Treatment to Prevent Heart Attack Trial. Metabolic and clinical outcomes in nondiabetic individuals with the metabolic syndrome assigned to chlorthalidone, amlodipine, or lisinopril as initial treatment for hypertension: a report from the Antihypertensive and Lipid-Lowering Treatment to Prevent Heart Attack Trial (ALLHAT). *Diabetes Care* 31:353–360.

Brenner BM, Cooper ME, de Zeeuw D, Keane WF, Mitch WE, Parving HH, Remuzzi G, Snapinn SM, Zhang Z, Shahinfar S; RENAAL Study Investigators (2001) Effects of losartan on renal and cardio-vascular outcomes in patients with type 2 diabetes and nephropathy. *N Engl J Med* 345:861–869.

Brownlee M (2005) The pathobiology of diabetic complications: a unifying mechanism. *Diabetes* 54:1615–1625.

Campbell S, Reeves D, Kontopantelis E, Middleton E, Sibbald B, Roland M (2007) Quality of primary care in England with the introduction of pay for performance. *N Engl J Med* 357:181–190.

Colhoun HM, Betteridge DJ, Durrington PN, Hitman GA, Neil HA, Livingstone SJ, Thomason MJ, Mackness MI, Charlton-Menys V, Fuller JH; CARDS Investigators (2004) Primary prevention of cardio-vascular disease with atorvastatin in type 2 diabetes in the Collaborative Atorvastatin Diabetes Study (CARDS): multicentre randomised placebo-controlled trial. *Lancet* 364:685–696.

Dahlöf B, Devereux RB, Kjeldsen SE, Julius S, Beevers G, de Faire U, Fyhrquist F, Ibsen H, Kristiansson K, Lederballe-Pedersen O, Lindholm LH, Nieminen MS, Omvik P, Oparil S, Wedel H; LIFE Study Group (2002) Cardiovascular morbidity and mortality in the Losartan Intervention For Endpoint reduction in hypertension study (LIFE): a randomised trial against atenolol. *Lancet* 359:995–1003.

Dahlöf B, Sever PS, Poulter NR, Wedel H, Beevers DG, Caulfield M, Collins R, Kjeldsen SE, Kristinsson A, McInnes GT, Mehlsen J, Nieminen M, O'Brien E, Ostergren J; ASCOT Investigators (2005) Prevention of cardiovascular events with an antihypertensive regimen of amlodipine adding perindopril as required versus atenolol adding bendroflumethiazide as required, in the Anglo-Scandinavian Cardiac Outcomes Trial–Blood Pressure Lowering Arm (ASCOT–BPLA): a multicentre randomised controlled trial. *Lancet* 366:895–906.

DCCT Research Group (1993) The effect of intensive treatment of diabetes on the development and progression of long-term complications in insulin-dependent diabetes mellitus. The Diabetes Control and Complications Trial Research Group. *N Engl J Med* 329:977–986.

De Block CE, Van Gaal LF (2009) GLP-1 receptor agonists for type 2 diabetes. *Lancet* **374**:4–6.

Deckert T, Feldt-Rasmussen B, Borch-Johnsen K, Jensen T, Kofoed-Enevoldsen A (1989) Albuminuria reflects widespread vascular damage. The Steno hypothesis. *Diabetologia* **32**:219–226.

Defronzo RA (2009) Banting Lecture. From the triumvirate to the ominous octet: a new paradigm for the treatment of type 2 diabetes mellitus. *Diabetes* **58**:773–795.

Dluhy RG, McMahon GT (2008) Intensive glycemic control in the ACCORD and ADVANCE trials. *N Engl J Med* **358**:2630–2633.

Duckworth W, Abraira C, Moritz T, Reda D, Emanuele N, Reaven PD, Zieve FJ, Marks J, Davis SN, Hayward R, Warren SR, Goldman S, McCarren M, Vitek ME, Henderson WG, Huang GD; VADT Investigators (2009) Glucose control and vascular complications in veterans with type 2 diabetes. *N Engl J Med* **360**:129–139.

ETDRS Research Group (1991) Effects of aspirin treatment on diabetic retinopathy. Early Treatment Diabetic Retinopathy Study report number 8. *Ophthalmology* **98**:757–765.

Fong DS, Aiello L, Gardner TW, King GL, Blankenship G, Cavallerano JD, Ferris FL, Klein R (2004) Retinopathy in diabetes. *Diabetes Care* **27**:S84–S87.

Funnell MM, Brown TL, Childs BP, Haas LB, Hosey GM, Jensen B, Maryniuk M, Peyrot M, Piette JD, Reader D, Siminerio LM, Weinger K, Weiss MA (2007) National standards for diabetes self-management education. *Diabetes Care* **30**:S96–S103.

Gaede P, Vedel P, Larsen N, Jensen GV, Parving HH, Pedersen O (2003) Multifactorial intervention and cardiovascular disease in patients with type 2 diabetes. *N Engl J Med* **348**:383–393.

Goldberg RB, Mellies MJ, Sacks FM, Moyé LA, Howard BV, Howard WJ, Davis BR, Cole TG, Pfeffer MA, Braunwald E; CARE Investigators (1998) Cardiovascular events and their reduction with pravastatin in diabetic and glucose-intolerant myocardial infarction survivors with average cholesterol levels: subgroup analyses in the cholesterol and recurrent events (CARE) trial. *Circulation* **98**:2513–2519.

Hansson L, Zanchetti A, Carruthers SG, Dahlöf B, Elmfeldt D, Julius S, Ménard J, Rahn KH, Wedel H, Westerling S (1998) Effects of intensive blood-pressure lowering and low-dose aspirin in patients with hypertension: principal results of the Hypertension Optimal Treatment (HOT) randomised trial. HOT Study Group. *Lancet* **351**:1755–1762.

Heart Outcomes Prevention Evaluation Study Investigators (2000) Effects of ramipril on cardiovascular and microvascular outcomes in people with diabetes mellitus: results of the HOPE study and MICRO–HOPE substudy. *Lancet* **355**:253–259.

Holman RR, Farmer AJ, Davies MJ, Levy JC, Darbyshire JL, Keenan JF, Paul SK; 4-T Study Group (2009) Three-year efficacy of complex insulin regimens in type 2 diabetes. *N Engl J Med* **361**:1736–1747.

Holman RR, Paul SK, Bethel MA, Matthews DR, Neil HA (2008) 10-year follow-up of intensive glucose control in type 2 diabetes. *N Engl J Med* **359**:1577–1578.

Keech A, Colquhoun D, Best J, Kirby A, Simes RJ, Hunt D, Hague W, Beller E, Arulchelvam M, Baker J, Tonkin A; LIPID Study Group (2003) Secondary prevention of cardiovascular events with long-term pravastatin in patients with diabetes or impaired fasting glucose: results from the LIPID trial. *Diabetes Care* **26**:2713–2721.

Kleiman NS, Lincoff AM, Kereiakes DJ, Miller DP, Aguirre FV, Anderson KM, Weisman HF, Califf RM, Topol EJ; EPILOG Investigators (1998) Diabetes mellitus, glycoprotein IIb/IIIa blockade, and heparin: evidence for a complex interaction in a multicenter trial. *Circulation* **97**:1912–1920.

Landon MB, Spong CY, Thom E, Carpenter MW, Ramin SM, Casey B, Wapner RJ, Varner MW, Rouse DJ, Thorp JM Jr, Sciscione A, Catalano P, Harper M, Saade G, Lain KY, Sorokin Y, Peaceman AM, Tolosa JE, Anderson GB; Eunice Kennedy Shriver National Institute of Child Health and Human Development Maternal-Fetal Medicine Units Network (2009) A multicenter, randomized trial of treatment for mild gestational diabetes. *N Engl J Med* **361**:1339–1348.

Leslie RD, Delli Castelli M (2004) Age-dependent influences on the origins of autoimmune diabetes: evidence and implications. *Diabetes* **53**:3033–3040.

Leslie RD (2010) Predicting adult-onset autoimmune diabetes: clarity from complexity. *Diabetes* **59**:330–331.

Lewis EJ, Hunsicker LG, Clarke WR, Berl T, Pohl MA, Lewis JB, Ritz E, Atkins RC, Rohde R, Raz I; Collaborative Study Group (2001) Renoprotective effect of the angiotensin-receptor antagonist irbesartan in patients with nephropathy due to type 2 diabetes. *N Engl J Med* **345**:851–860.

Malmberg K, Rydén L, Efendic S, Herlitz J, Nicol P, Waldenström A, Wedel H, Welin L (1995) Randomized trial of insulin-glucose infusion followed by subcutaneous insulin treatment in diabetic patients with acute myocardial infarction (DIGAMI study): effects on mortality at 1 year. *J Am Coll Cardiol* **26**:57–65.

Malmberg K, Rydén L, Wedel H, Birkeland K, Bootsma A, Dickstein K, Efendic S, Fisher M, Hamsten A, Herlitz J, Hildebrandt P, MacLeod K, Laakso M, Torp-Pedersen C, Waldenström A; DIGAMI 2 Investigators (2005) Intense metabolic control by means of insulin in patients with diabetes mellitus and acute myocardial infarction (DIGAMI 2): effects on mortality and morbidity. *Eur Heart J* **26**:650–661.

Marso SP, Lincoff AM, Ellis SG, Bhatt DL, Tanguay JF, Kleiman NS, Hammoud T, Booth JE, Sapp SK, Topol EJ (1999) Optimizing the percutaneous interventional outcomes for patients with diabetes mellitus: results of the EPISTENT (Evaluation of platelet IIb/IIIa inhibitor for stenting trial) diabetic substudy. *Circulation* **100**:2477–2484.

Murphy R, Ellard S, Hattersley AT (2008) Clinical implications of a molecular genetic classification of monogenic beta-cell diabetes. *Nat Clin Pract Endocrinol Metab* **4**:200–213.

Naik RG, Brooks-Worrell BM, Palmer JP (2009) Latent autoimmune diabetes in adults. *J Clin Endocrinol Metab* **94**:4635–4644.

Nathan DM, Cleary PA, Backlund JY, Genuth SM, Lachin JM, Orchard TJ, Raskin P, Zinman B; Diabetes Control and Complications Trial/ Epidemiology of Diabetes Interventions and Complications (DCCT/EDIC) Study Research Group (2005) Intensive diabetes treatment and cardiovascular disease in patients with type 1 diabetes. *N Engl J Med* **353**:2643–2653.

Ohkubo Y, Kishikawa H, Araki E, Miyata T, Isami S, Motoyoshi S, Kojima Y, Furuyoshi N, Shichiri M (1995) Intensive insulin therapy prevents the progression of diabetic microvascular complications in Japanese patients with non-insulin-dependent diabetes mellitus: a randomized prospective 6-year study. *Diabetes Res Clin Pract* **28**:103–117.

Parving H-H, Lehnert H, Brochner-Mortensen J, Gomis R, Andersen S, Arner P (2001) The effect of irbesartan on the development of diabetic nephropathy in patients with type 2 diabetes. *N Engl J Med* **345**:870–878.

Rowan JA, Hague WM, Gao W, Battin MR, Moore MP; MiG Trial Investigators (2008) Metformin versus insulin for the treatment of gestational diabetes. *N Engl J Med* **358**:2003–2015.

Rubins HB, Robins SJ, Collins D, Nelson DB, Elam MB, Schaefer EJ, Faas FH, Anderson JW (2002) Diabetes, plasma insulin, and cardiovascular disease: subgroup analysis from the Department of Veterans Affairs high-density lipoprotein intervention trial (VA-HIT). *Arch Intern Med* **162**:2597–2604.

Ruggenenti P, Fassi A, Ilieva AP, Bruno S, Iliev IP, Brusegan V, Rubis N, Gherardi G, Arnoldi F, Ganeva M, Ene-Iordache B, Gaspari F, Perna A, Bossi A, Trevisan R, Dodesini AR, Remuzzi G; Bergamo Nephrologic Diabetes Complications Trial (BENEDICT) Investigators (2004) Preventing microalbuminuria in type 2 diabetes. *N Engl J Med* **351**:1941–1951.

Schauer PR, Kashyap SR, Wolski K, Brethauer SA, Kirwan JP, Pothier CE, Thomas S, Abood B, Nissen SE, Bhatt DL (2012) Bariatric surgery versus intensive medical therapy in obese patients with diabetes. *N Engl J Med* **366**:1567–1576.

Sever PS, Poulter NR, Dahlöf B, Wedel H, Collins R, Beevers G, Caulfield M, Kjeldsen SE, Kristinsson A, McInnes GT, Mehlsen J, Nieminen M, O'Brien E, Ostergren J (2005) Reduction in cardiovascular events with atorvastatin in 2,532 patients with type 2 diabetes: Anglo-Scandinavian Cardiac Outcomes Trial – lipid-lowering arm (ASCOT-LLA). *Diabetes Care* **28**:1151–1157.

UKPDS Group (1998) Intensive blood-glucose control with sulphonylureas or insulin compared with conventional treatment and risk of complications in patients with type 2 diabetes (UKPDS 33). *Lancet* **352**:837–853.

UKPDS Group (1998) Tight blood pressure control and risk of macrovascular and microvascular complications in type 2 diabetes (UKPDS 38). *BMJ* **317**:703–713.

Umpierrez GE, Smiley D, Jacobs S, Peng L, Temponi A, Mulligan P, Umpierrez D, Newton C, Olson D, Rizzo M (2011) Randomized study of basal–bolus insulin therapy in the inpatient management of patients with type 2 diabetes undergoing general surgery (RABBIT 2 surgery). *Diabetes Care* **34**:256–261.

Whelton PK, Barzilay J, Cushman WC, Davis BR, Iiamathi E, Kostis JB, Leenen FH, Louis GT, Margolis KL, Mathis DE, Moloo J, Nwachuku C, Panebianco D, Parish DC, Pressel S, Simmons DL, Thadani U; ALLHAT Collaborative Research Group (2005) Clinical outcomes in antihypertensive treatment of type 2 diabetes, impaired fasting glucose concentration, and normoglycemia: Antihypertensive and Lipid-Lowering Treatment to Prevent Heart Attack Trial (ALLHAT). *Arch Intern Med* **165**:1401–1409.

Resources

Research and support organizations

American Diabetes Association
Center for Information
1701 North Beauregard Street
Alexandria, VA 22311
USA

Website: www.diabetes.org

Dose Adjustment For Normal Eating (DAFNE)
Central DAFNE Administration Office
Diabetes Resources Centre
North Tyneside General Hospital
Rake Lane
North Shields, Tyne and Wear
NE29 8NH
UK

Website: www.dafne.uk.com

European Association for the Study of Diabetes (EASD)
Rheindorfer Weg 3
40591 Düsseldorf
Germany

Website: www.easd.org
Email: secretariat@easd.org

European Foundation for the Study of Diabetes (EFSD)
Rheindorfer Weg 3
40591 Düsseldorf
Germany

Website: www.europeandiabetesfoundation.org
Email: foundation@easd.org

Foundation of European Nurses in Diabetes (FEND)
37 Earls Drive
Newcastle on Tyne
NE15 7AL
UK

Website: www.fend.org

International Diabetes Federation (IDF)
166 Chaussée de la Hulpe
B-1170 Brussels
Belgium

Website: http://www.idf.org/
Email : info@idf.org

International Society for Paediatric and Adolescent Diabetes (ISPAD)
c/o KIT, Kurfürstendamm 71
10709 Berlin
Germany

Website: www.ispad.org
Email:secretariat@ispad.org

JDRF (formerly Juvenile Diabetes Research Foundation)
JDRF London
19 Angel Gate
City Road
London
EC1V 2PT
UK

Website: www.jdrf.org.uk
Email: info@jdrf.org.uk

JDRF USA
26 Broadway
New York
NY 10004
USA

Website: www.jdrf.org
E-mail: info@jdrf.org/

National Institute for Health and Clinical Excellence (NICE)
MidCity Place
71 High Holborn
London
WC1V 6NA
UK

Website: www.nice.org.uk
Email: nice@nice.org.uk

World Diabetes Foundation (WDF)
Brogårdsvej 70
DK-2820 Gentofte
Denmark
Website: www.worlddiabetesfoundation.org

World Health Organization (WHO)
Avenue Appia 2
1211 Geneva 27
Switzerland
Website: www.who.int
Email: info@who.int

Selected regional and national diabetes association websites

Africa
IDF African Regional Office: www.idf-africa.org
Diabetes Kenya Association: www.diabeteskenya.org
Diabetes South Africa: www.diabetessa.co.za
Tanzania Diabetes Association: www.tanzaniadiabetes-association.org

Europe
IDF European Regional Office: www.idf-europe.org
Austrian Diabetes Organization: www.diabetes.or.at
Belgian Diabetes Association: www.diabete-abd.be
Flemish Diabetes Association: www.diabetes-vdv.be
Danish Diabetes Association: www.diabetes.dk
Finnish Diabetes Association: www.diabetes.fi
French Diabetes Association: www.afd.asso.fr
German Diabetes Association: www.diabetesunion.de
Hellenic Diabetes Association: www.ede.gr
Hungarian Diabetes Association: www.diabet.hu
Icelandic Diabetes Association: www.diabetes.is
Diabetes Federation of Ireland: www.diabetes.ie
Israel Diabetes Association: www.sukeret.co.il
Italian Diabetes Association: www.assitdiab.it
Lithuania Diabetes Association: www.is.it/diabetas
Luxembourg Diabetes Association: www.ald.lu
Maltese Diabetes Association: www.diabetesmalta.org
Netherlands Diabetes Association: www.diabetesverening.nl
Norwegian Diabetes Association: www.diabetes.no
Polish Diabetic Association: www.diabetyk.org.pl
Portuguese Diabetic Association: www.apdp.pt
Russian Diabetes Federation: www.rda.org.ru
Slovak Diabetic Society: www.diadays-tn.sk
Slovenia Diabetes Association: www.diabetes-zveza.si
Spanish Diabetic Society: www.sediabetes.org
Swedish Diabetes Association: www.diabetes.se
Swiss Diabetes Association: www.diabetesgesellschaft.ch
Turkish Diabetes Foundation: www.turdiab.org
Diabetes UK: www.diabetes.org.uk
European Association for the Study of Diabetes (EASD): www.easd.org

Middle East and North Africa
IDF MENA Regional Office: www.idf-mena.org
Iranian Diabetes Society: www.ir-diabetes-society.com
Jordanian Society for the Care of Diabetes: www.jscd.jo
Saudi Diabetes and Endocrine Association: www.sdea.org.sa
Qatar Diabetes Association: www.qda.org.qa

North America and Caribbean
IDF NAC Regional Office: www.idf-nac.org
American Diabetes Association: www.diabetes.org
Canada Diabetes Association: www.diabetes.ca
Diabète Québec: www.diabete.qc.ca
International Chair on Cardiometabolic Risk: www.cardiometabolic-risk.org

South and Central America
IDF SACA Regional Office: www.idf-saca.org
Argentine League for the Protection of Diabetics: www.diabetesaldia.com
Argentinian Diabetes Society: www.diabetes.org.ar
Associacão de Diabetes Juvenil, Brazil: www.adj.org.br
Federcão Nacional de Associacões de Diabéticos (FENAD): www.anad.org.br
Brazilian Diabetes Society: www.diabetes.org.br
Patronato de Pacientes Diabéticos de Guatemala: http://www.diabetes.com.gt
Asociación Puertorriqueña de Diabetes: www.diabetespr.org
Asociación de Diabéticos del Uruguay: www.adu.org.uy

Southeast Asia
IDF SEA Regional Office: www.idf-sea.org
Diabetic Association of Bangladesh: www.dab-bd.org
Diabetic Association of India:www.dairaheja.org
Diabetic Association of Sri Lanka: www.diabetessrilanka.org

Western Pacific
IDF Western Pacific Regional Office: www.idf-wp.org
Diabetes Australia: www.diabetesaustralia.com.au
Diabetes Hong Kong: www.diabetes-hk.org
Japan Diabetes Society: www.jds.or.jp
Diabetes New Zealand: www.diabetes.org.nz
Philippine Diabetes Association: www.diabetesphil.org
Diabetes Society of Singapore: www.dss.org.sg

Glossary

A

Accelerator hypothesis This proposes that the onset of type 1 diabetes occurs earlier in those with insulin resistance or heavier weight (i.e. with predisposition to type 2 diabetes).

Adenosine triphosphate (ATP) A coenzyme used in the intracellular metabolism of energy.

Adiponectin A cytokine derived from adipocytes that is associated with improved glycemic control and lipid profiles in patients with diabetes.

Advanced glycation end-product (AGE) Formed when excess glucose combines nonenzymatically with tissue or circulating proteins. AGEs are increased in diabetes, and contribute to microvascular complications.

Aldose reductase Some of the glucose that enters the cell is metabolized by this enzyme into sorbitol, which in turn is implicated as a factor for some microvascular complications.

Allele One of a pair of genes found in a specific location on a chromosome.

Alpha-glucosidase inhibitors A class of diabetes drugs that decrease intestinal absorption of glucose by inhibiting the breakdown of carbohydrates into monosaccharides in the small bowel.

Amylin An amino acid stored in the beta cells of the pancreas and co-secreted with insulin, that can decrease postprandial glucagon, increase satiety and slow down gastric emptying.

Angiotensin-converting enzyme inhibitors (ACEIs) A class of drugs that inhibit the conversion of angiotensin I into angiotensin II – a vasoconstrictor. ACEIs also inhibit kininases – enzymes that inactivate kinins (plasma proteins important in vasodilation).

Angiotensin receptor blockers (ARBs) A class of drugs that block the action of angiotensin II on the type 1 angiotensin II receptor, resulting in vasodilation and decreased blood pressure.

Atherosclerosis Thickening of the arterial wall as a result of fat deposition. Patients with diabetes have accelerated atherosclerotic vascular disease.

Autoantibody An antibody that reacts to the patient's own cells or tissues. Islet cell autoantibodies are strongly associated with the development of type 1 diabetes.

Autoantigen An antigen that is present in the endogenous tissue, and stimulates the production of antibodies (autoantibodies).

Autonomic neuropathy Damage of the nerves that are not in the patient's conscious control (such as nerves of the cardiovascular, gastrointestinal and genitourinary systems).

B

Bariatric surgery Surgery to promote weight loss by altering the gastrointestinal anatomy.

Basal–bolus insulin secretion The physiological pattern of insulin secretion whereby a relatively constant amount of insulin is secreted in the fasting state, and a rise in insulin secretion is seen in response to meals.

Beta cell A type of cell located in the pancreatic islet of Langerhans that produces insulin and amylin. Type 1 diabetes is caused by the autoimmune destruction or dysfunction of most of the β cells, while in type 2 diabetes they fail gradually over time.

Body mass index (BMI) A measurement to estimate body fat, calculated by dividing a person's weight in kilograms by their height in square meters (kg/m^2). A BMI of less than 18 is considered underweight, 18 to 24.9 is normal, 25 to 29.9 is overweight, and 30 and above is obese.

Brittle diabetes Diabetes with labile blood glucoses and episodes of hypoglycemia and/or ketoacidosis.

C

Calcium channel A voltage-gated ion channel on the cell membrane, the opening of which allows calcium to enter the cell, with resultant release of insulin.

Charcot's arthropathy Deformity of the foot resulting from sensory neuropathy, the most common cause of which is diabetes.

C-peptide In humans, proinsulin is cleaved into C-peptide and insulin. C-peptide can be used as an indicator of beta-cell function or insulin secretion.

Creatinine A metabolic by-product of creatine, an amino acid found in muscle. The creatinine blood level is used to measure kidney function.

D

Dawn phenomenon An increase in blood glucoses in the early morning, thought to be a result of a rise in counterregulatory hormones (cortisol, catecholamines and growth hormone).

Diabetes insipidus A disorder of the posterior pituitary gland that leads to decreased levels of anti-diuretic hormone, resulting in polyuria and polydipsia.

Diabetic ketoacidosis (DKA) Severe metabolic disturbance seen in diabetes, consisting of a triad of hyperglycemia, ketonemia, and anion gap acidosis.

Dipeptidyl peptidase-4 (DPP-4) inhibitors A class of diabetes drugs that inhibit dipeptidyl peptidase-4, the enzyme that degrades glucagon-like peptide-1 (GLP-1). This results in lowering of glucose levels, especially during the mealtime excursions.

Double diabetes Diabetes with features of both type 1 and type 2 diabetes.

Dyslipidemia Derangement in lipid (cholesterol and triglyceride) levels and composition. Dyslipidemia contributes to atherosclerosis.

E

Enteroinsular axis The physiologic pathway involving the intestinal hormones (incretins) and pancreatic hormones (insulin, glucagon) that leads to glucose homeostasis.

Epithelium A layer of cells that line the cavities and surfaces of structures throughout the body.

F

Fasting plasma glucose (FPG) A measurement of plasma glucose in the morning (typically around 8 am) after fasting for at least 8 hours overnight.

Free fatty acids (FFA) Also known as non-esterified fatty acids (NEFA), these are long-chain (typically 14–18 carbon atoms) carboxylic acids, which are one of the main forms of lipid in the circulation, used by the body as fuel. NEFA molecules may be of different chain lengths and be saturated or unsaturated. Elevated plasma levels of FFA are a major cause of insulin resistance in the liver and skeletal muscle.

G

Gestational diabetes mellitus (GDM) Elevation of plasma glucose to diabetic levels, occurring during the course of a pregnancy and typically remitting after the pregnancy.

Glomerular filtration rate (GFR) The volume of blood flow per minute through the renal glomeruli.

Glucagon A hormone produced by the alpha cells of the islets of Langerhans; it has generally anti-insulin effects and forms part of the feedback loop that stabilizes glucose levels.

Glucagon-like peptide-1 (GLP-1) A hormone released from the L cells of the distal end of the small bowel and the proximal end of the large bowel, usually in response to eating.

Glucokinase An enzyme that facilitates phosphory-lation of glucose to glucose-6-phosphate.

Gluconeogenesis The synthesis of glucose from non-carbohydrate substrates, such as amino acids and fatty acids.

Glucose A simple carbohydrate (monosaccharide), $C_6H_{12}O_6$, used by cells as the primary source of energy.

Glucose intolerance Abnormally high levels of plasma glucose, defined after oral ingestion of (75 g) glucose; typically refers to levels above normal but less than would define diabetes.

Glucose transporter (GLUT) One of a group of membrane proteins that facilitate the transport of glucose across tissue membranes.

Glucotoxicity/glycotoxicity Adverse effects ascribed to persistent elevation of plasma glucose.

Glycemic index (GI) An estimation of the extent to which a specific foodstuff will elevate plasma glucose; sometimes taken to refer specifically to the carbohydrate content of the foodstuff.

Glycogen A polysaccharide; the principal storage form of glucose in humans, found mainly in the liver and muscles.

Glycogenesis The process of glycogen synthesis from glucose.

Glycogenolysis The process of breakdown of glycogen to glucose.

Glycolysis The intracellular metabolic pathway that converts glucose into high-energy compounds, prin-cipally ATP.

Glycosuria The presence of glucose in the urine. This is usually indicative of impaired glucose tolerance or diabetes.

H

Hemoglobin A1c (HbA1c/glycated hemoglobin) A form of hemoglobin to which glucose is bound; now universally accepted as a useful clinical measure of long-term glycemic control in diabetes.

High-density lipoproteins (HDL) Circulating lipoproteins of density >1.063 g/ml, that collect cholesterol from the tissues and return it to the liver, where it is metabolized and excreted, and to the adrenal glands and gonads for synthesis of steroid hormones. HDL are sometimes referred to as the 'good cholesterol' lipoproteins.

Histocompatibility leukocyte antigen (HLA) The major histocompatibility complex (MHC) in human chromosomes, it comprises a number of genes related to immune function, such as rejection of foreign tissue and expression of autoimmune disease.

Hyperglycemia Excessive levels of glucose in the blood plasma.

Hyperinsulinemia Excessive levels of insulin in the blood relative to the level of glucose.

Hyperosmolality Increased concentration of solutes in a body fluid, e.g. blood, expressed as osmoles of solute per kilogram of serum.

Hyperosmolar nonketotic hyperglycemia (HONK) Also known as hyperosmolar hyper-glycemic state (HHS), this condition is seen more often in type 2 than in type 1 diabetes. It is associated with extremely high plasma glucose, raised urea, electrolyte disturbance, and severe dehydration.

Hypoglycemia An abnormally low level of plasma glucose and a common complication of insulin treatment. Hypoglycemia results from an imbalance between injected insulin or oral therapy and a patient's diet, activity, and metabolic requirements.

I

Impaired glucose tolerance (IGT) An abnormal glycemic state, defined as a plasma glucose level of 140 to 199 mg/dl (7.8 to 11.1 mmol/l) 2 hours after the oral ingestion of 75 g of glucose; frequently a precursor to the development of type 2 diabetes.

Incidence A measurement of the number of new individuals who contract a disease during a particular period of time. Usually expressed as the number of cases per year per population. *See also* prevalence.

Incretin effect The greater increase in plasma insulin occurring after oral ingestion of glucose compared to the rise seen after the same amount given intravenously. It is caused by the release of gut hormones known as incretins, and accounts for probably 50–70% of the insulin rise.

Insulin A hormone produced by the β cells of the islets of Langerhans that is the principal hormone regulating glucose, but is also important in regulating fat and carbohydrate metabolism.

Insulin analog An altered, synthetic form of insulin, in which certain amino acids are modified to affect the time course of the insulin action.

Insulin deficiency Inability to produce sufficient insulin; the state of having insufficient insulin relative to the prevailing glucose level.

Insulin-like growth factor (IGF) A protein with a structure similar to insulin, and that may interact with insulin receptors and share some actions with insulin.

Insulin receptor A cell membrane receptor activated by insulin to initiate a signaling cascade that stimulates glucose uptake.

Insulin resistance A condition in which cells and tissues respond suboptimally to insulin stimulation. Untreated insulin resistance can lead to type 2 diabetes.

Insulin secretagogue A substance which stimulates the secretion of insulin from the pancreas. Sulfonyl-ureas, repaglinide, and nateglinide are all in this category of drugs.

Insulin sensitivity A measure of how well an individual responds to insulin.

Intraretinal microvascular abnormality (IRMA) A very small abnormality of the retinal blood vessels, representing or serving as a precursor to new vessel formation.

Islets of Langerhans The endocrine tissue of the pancreas, containing alpha, beta, and delta cells; they are discrete microscopic 'islands' of tissue scattered throughout the pancreas, and the source of insulin, glucagon, and other hormones.

K

Ketoacidosis A metabolic acidosis with the organic acid forms of ketone bodies as the major anions involved. *See also* diabetic ketoacidosis.

Ketone/ketone body One of a family of organic ketones or their organic acid forms, namely aceto-acetate, β-hydroxybutyrate, or acetate.

L

Lactic acidosis A metabolic acidosis with lactic acid as the major anion involved.

Latent autoimmune diabetes of adults (LADA) A slow-onset form of diabetes occurring in adults, closely related to type 1 diabetes.

Leptin A hormone released almost entirely from white adipose tissue, its absence causes insatiable hunger, reduction in metabolic rate, and infertility, among other effects.

Lipoatrophy Atrophy of adipose tissue, which can have a variety of causes, including subcutaneous insulin injection.

Lipohypertrophy Hypertrophy of adipose tissue, usually as a consequence of chronic local insulin injection.

Lipolysis Breakdown of fat, usually triglyceride, which can be either circulating or intracellular.

Lipoprotein A spherical structure composed of lipids and proteins surrounding a core of cholesterol and triglycerides, used to transport these fats through the bloodstream. They can be classified according to density, of which there are five types: chylomicrons; very-low-density lipoproteins (VLDL); intermediate-density lipoproteins (IDL); low-density lipoproteins (LDL); high-density lipoproteins (HDL). *See also* individual types.

Lipotoxicity The concept that excess availability of lipid (which may be of several forms) inhibits normal function of glucoregulatory mechanisms.

Low-density lipoproteins (LDL) Circulating lipoproteins of density 1.019–1.063 g/ml that transport cholesterol from the liver to the tissues. Cholesterol carried in LDL particles is especially atherogenic and hence these are colloquially called 'bad cholesterol' lipoproteins.

M

Macroalbuminuria Albuminuria of sufficient degree to be detectable with routine urine testing strips (>300 mg/24 hr or >300 mg/l on a spot sample).

Macrosomia Also known as 'big baby syndrome' or 'large for gestational age', macrosomia describes excessive intra-uterine growth. In neonates, it is usually defined as a weight of more than 4000–4500 g.

Maculopathy A pathological condition of the macula (the area of the retina specialized for high acuity vision), particularly that caused by diabetic retinopathy.

Major histocompatibility complex (MHC) A group of cell-surface molecules that mediate cell interactions with the immune system.

Maturity onset diabetes of the young (MODY) A group of forms of diabetes that are strongly hered-itable – usually as autosomal dominant traits – that occur typically before mid-life, but not requiring insulin.

Metabolic syndrome A group of co-segregating medical disorders that independently or together increase the risk of developing cardiovascular disease and diabetes. Defining criteria include central obesity, dyslipidemia, raised BP, raised FPG, microalbumin-uria, and hypertension.

Metformin A biguanide drug, now the first-line therapy for type 2 diabetes.

Michaelis constant (abbreviated K_m) The substrate concentration at which a reaction obeying Michaelis–Menton kinetics (a model which describes the rate of enzymatic reactions) is at half-maximum rate. Different K_m values of different glucose transporters (GLUTs) enable specific functions.

Microalbuminuria Albuminuria of modest degree, not detectable with routine urine testing strips (<300 mg/l on a spot sample).

Mononeuritis multiplex Damage to one or more peripheral nerves occurring within a relatively short time.

Mononeuropathy Damage to a single nerve or nerve group, which results in loss of movement, sensation, or other function of that nerve.

N

Neuroglycopenia The consequences of a shortage of glucose supply to the brain, usually caused by severe hypoglycemia.

Nonesterified fatty acids (NEFA) *See* free fatty acids (FFA).

Nonproliferative diabetic retinopathy (NPDR) The earliest stage of diabetic retinopathy, in which damaged blood vessels in the retina begin to leak fluid and small amounts of blood into the back of the eye.

Nephropathy Kidney damage, caused in diabetes by glomerular and vascular changes.

Neuropathy Nerve damage, possibly caused in diabetes by microvascular injury. Diabetic neuro-pathy can affect peripheral nerves, autonomic nerves and cranial nerves.

O

Osmolal gap The difference between measured serum osmolality and calculated serum osmolarity, usually <10 mOsm/kg, but may be increased by large amounts of alcohols, proteins or unmeasured sugar (e.g. mannose).

Osmolality, serum A measure of electrolyte–water balance, estimated as the amount of dissoved chemicals (notably sodium, potassium, glucose and urea) in a given volume of blood serum; it is measured in osmoles (Osm) of solute per kilogram of solvent (Osm/kg).

Osmolarity Very similar in clinical relevance to osmolality, it is a measure of the osmoles of solute per liter of solution (osmol/l or Osm/l).

Osteomyelitis Acute or chronic bone infection; one of a range of foot complications affecting diabetic patients.

Oxidative stress An imbalance between reactive oxygen species and a biological system's ability to detoxify the reactive intermediates or to repair the resulting damage. The term has no close, or agreed, definition.

P

Peripheral arterial disease (PAD) A disease associated with atherosclerosis in those peripheral arteries that carry blood to the body and especially – in disease terms – to the head and limbs.

Peroxisome proliferative-activated receptor (PPAR) One of a group of receptor proteins, found in the cell nucleus, which activate the transcription of the genes that regulate cell differentiation, function, and metabolism – notably the response to insulin stimulus.

Polydipsia Excessive thirst; a clinical hallmark of hyperglycemia.

Polyphagia Excessive hunger/appetite due to poor glucose metabolism.

Polyuria Excessive production or passage of urine (at least 2.5 or 3.0 l over 24 hours in adults). Polyuria is a typical clinical feature of high blood glucose due to diabetes.

Potassium channel An ion channel on the cell membrane that allows potassium to pass into and out of the cell. ATP-gated potassium channels are important in the secretion of insulin and the action of sulfonylureas.

Pre-eclampsia A condition associated with both hypertension which arises in pregnancy (pregnancy-induced hypertension) and with significant amounts of protein in the urine; it is a dangerous complication with risk to both mother and baby.

Prevalence A measurement of the total (as distinct from new) number of cases in a population at a given time. It can be used to estimate how common a condition is. Sometimes given as 'lifetime prevalence', if referring to individuals who have had a diagnosis at some point in their lives, or 'current prevalence' to describe the percentage of people who currently have a diagnosis. *See also* incidence.

Proinsulin The prohormone precursor to insulin, which is converted inside the insulin-secreting cells to insulin and C-peptide.

Proliferative diabetic retinopathy (PDR) A serious complication of diabetes. Ischemic damage to the retinal blood vessels leads to the secretion of growth factors which cause abnormal blood vessels to grow on the surface of the retina (neovascularization). These new vessels are fragile and prone to hemorrhage; blindness can result.

Protein kinase C-beta (PKC-β) One of a family of protein kinase enzymes that modify other proteins through the addition of a phosphate group to one of the amino acids. This phosphorylation usually effects a functional change in the target protein. Activation of PKC-β by high intracellular glucose affects vasoconstriction, for instance.

Proteinuria The presence of serum proteins in the urine; this is a hallmark of diabetic kidney disease, especially when there is no blood in the urine.

Pyelonephritis An ascending urinary tract infection that has reached the renal pelvis or pyelum to cause inflammation of the kidney; also referred to as pyelitis.

R

Reactive oxygen species (ROS) Chemically reactive molecules containing oxygen, generated as by-products of cellular metabolism. High intracellular glucose causes increased ROS production, leading to oxidative stress and cell damage.

S

Second messenger system Molecules that relay signals from intercellular (primary) messengers – such as hormones or neurotransmitters – from receptors on the cell surface to target molecules in the cytoplasm or nucleus.

Secondary diabetes A form of diabetes that develops as a result of another disease or condition. For example, endocrine diseases such as Cushing's disease, pancreatitis, and steroid therapy can each cause secondary diabetes.

Sensorimotor neuropathy A process that damages nerve cells, nerve fibers (axons), and nerve coverings (myelin sheath) so that nerve signals are less rapid. Nerves that supply sensation to the feet are often damaged in diabetes.

Sodium–glucose co-transporter (SGLT) One of a a family of glucose transporters found in the mucosa of the small intestine (SGLT1) and the proximal tubule of the nephron (SGLT2). SGLT2 plays an important role in renal glucose reabsorption and SGLT2 inhibitors represent a new strategy in antihyperglycemic therapy.

Sorbitol A polyol or sugar alcohol, occurring naturally in fruit and used as a sweetener in many foods. Sorbitol is converted to fructose in the liver, which is not dependent on insulin for metabolism. However, the process of oxidizing accumulated sorbitol in the cells, particularly those of the retina, can lead to intracellular damage.

Sudomotor dysfunction An abnormality of the sweat glands leading to inappropriate sweating. It is a feature of nerve damage in diabetes.

Sulfonylurea (SU) One of a class of glucose-lowering drugs that are used in the management of type 2 diabetes. They act by increasing insulin release from the pancreatic β cells through the activation of potassium channel receptors.

T

Thiazolidinedione (TZD) One of a class of drugs, also known as glitazones, used in the treatment of type 2 diabetes. They work by activating nuclear receptors (PPARs) to increase insulin sensitivity.

Triglyceride A single molecule of glycerol combined with three fatty acids, triglycerides are the principal type of fat stored in the body. High triglyceride levels in the blood tend to coexist with low levels of HDL, contributing to diabetic dyslipidemia, and are associated with an increased risk of atherosclerosis.

Type 1 diabetes A form of diabetes mellitus that results from autoimmune destruction of the insulin-producing β cells of the pancreas. The subsequent lack of insulin leads to increased blood and urine glucose and often, but not always, requires insulin treatment.

Type 1B diabetes Also referred to as idiopathic diabetes, or diabetes of unknown origin, this form of type 1 diabetes is not autoimmune in nature and may be due to a viral infection. People with type 1b have an acute onset of insulin deficiency and even ketoacidosis (due to very high blood glucose).

Type 2 diabetes A metabolic disorder that is characterized by high blood glucose in the context of decreased insulin sensitivity and relatively decreased insulin secretion. This is the most prevalent form of diabetes and largely accounts for the current global 'epidemic'.

U

Ulcer (ischemic/neuropathic foot)

A break in the skin leading to wounds or open sores. The result of peripheral neuropathy, peripheral arterial disease, and other factors, foot ulcers are an important complication of diabetes, as they may lead to infection and amputation.

V

Vagal neuropathy A condition in which the vagal nerve is damaged. The vagal nerve is involved in the function of several organs, notably the stomach and its acid production, so vagal neuropathy is associated with abnormal clearance of food from the gut.

Vascular endothelial growth factor (VEGF)

A signal protein that is produced by cells and stimulates the production of new blood vessels. It is part of the system that restores the oxygen supply to tissues when blood circulation is inadequate, but can lead to inappropriate new vessel formation in the eyes. *See also* retinopathy, proliferative diabetic.

Very-low-density lipoproteins (VLDL)

Circulating lipoproteins of density 0.95–1.006 g/ml that carry newly synthesized triglycerides from the liver to the adipose tissues. They break down in the bloodstream to become IDL and LDL.

Vitreous hemorrhage The leakage of blood into the vitreous humor of the eye – in diabetes, particularly from weak, new vessels – which can cause acute loss of vision. *See also* retinopathy, proliferative diabetic.

Index